Treatment of Complex Cervical Spine Disorders

Guest Editors

FRANK M. PHILLIPS, MD
SAFDAR N. KHAN, MD

ORTHOPEDIC CLINICS OF NORTH AMERICA

www.orthopedic.theclinics.com

January 2012 • Volume 43 • Number 1

SAUNDERS an imprint of ELSEVIER, Inc.

W.B. SAUNDERS COMPANY
A Division of Elsevier Inc.

1600 John F. Kennedy Blvd. • Suite 1800 • Philadelphia, PA 19103-2899.

http://www.orthopedic.theclinics.com

ORTHOPEDIC CLINICS OF NORTH AMERICA Volume 43, Number 1
January 2012 ISSN 0030-5898, ISBN-13: 978-1-4557-3904-2

Editor: David Parsons

Orthopedic Clinics of North America (ISSN 0030-5898) is published quarterly by Elsevier Inc., 360 Park Avenue South, New York, NY 10010-1710. Months of issue are January, April, July, and October. Business and Editorial Offices: 1600 John F. Kennedy Blvd., Suite 1800, Philadelphia, PA 19103-2899. Customer Service Office: 3251 Riverport Lane, Maryland Heights, MO 63043. Periodicals postage paid at New York, NY and additional mailing offices. Subscription prices are $293.00 per year for (US individuals), $554.00 per year for (US institutions), $347.00 per year (Canadian individuals), $664.00 per year (Canadian institutions), $427.00 per year (international individuals), $664.00 per year (international institutions), $144.00 per year (US students), $208.00 per year (Canadian and international students). Foreign air speed delivery is included in all *Clinics* subscription prices. All prices are subject to change without notice. **POSTMASTER: Send change of address to** *Orthopedic Clinics of North America,* **Elsevier Health Sciences Division, Subscription Customer Service, 3251 Riverport Lane, Maryland Heights, MO 63043. Customer Service (orders, claims, online, change of address): Elsevier Health Sciences Division, Subscription Customer Service, 3251 Riverport Lane, Maryland Heights, MO 63043. Tel: 1-800-654-2452 (U.S. and Canada); 314-447-8871 (outside U.S. and Canada). Fax: 314-447-8029. E-mail: journalscustomerservice-usa@elsevier. com (for print support); journalsonlinesupport-usa@elsevier.com (for online support).**

Reprints. For copies of 100 or more, of articles in this publication, please contact the Commercial Reprints Department, Elsevier Inc., 360 Park Avenue South, New York, NY 10010-1710. Tel.: 212-633-3812; Fax: 212-462-1935; E-mail: reprints@elsevier. com.

Orthopedic Clinics of North America is covered in *MEDLINE/PubMed (Index Medicus), Cinahl, Excerpta Medica,* and *Cumulative Index to Nursing and Allied Health Literature.*

Printed and bound by CPI Group (UK) Ltd, Croydon, CR0 4YY

Transferred to Digital Print 2012

Contributors

GUEST EDITORS

FRANK M. PHILLIPS, MD
Professor, Orthopaedic Surgery; Co-Director, Spine Fellowship, Rush University Medical Center, Chicago, Illinois

SAFDAR N. KHAN, MD
Assistant Professor, Department of Orthopaedics, The Ohio State University, Columbus, Ohio

AUTHORS

TODD J. ALBERT, MD
Richard H. Rothman Professor and Chairman, Department of Orthopaedic Surgery; Professor of Neurosurgery, Thomas Jefferson University and Hospitals; President, The Rothman Institute, Philadelphia, Pennsylvania

HOWARD S. AN, MD
Professor, Department of Orthopaedics, Rush University Medical Center, Chicago, Illinois

D. GREG ANDERSON, MD
Professor, Department of Orthopaedic Surgery, Rothman Institute, Thomas Jefferson University and Hospitals, Philadelphia, Pennsylvania

DARREL S. BRODKE, MD
Louis and Janet Peery Presidential Endowed Chair, Professor and Vice Chairman, Department of Orthopaedics, University of Utah, Salt Lake City, Utah

PAUL C. CELESTRE, MD
Resident Physician, Department of Orthopaedic Surgery, UCLA Comprehensive Spine Center, Santa Monica, California

CHRIS A. CORNETT, MD
Assistant Professor, Department of Orthopaedic Surgery and Rehabilitation, University of Nebraska Medical Center, Omaha, Nebraska

BRADFORD L. CURRIER, MD
Professor of Orthopedic Surgery, Consultant, Department of Orthopedic Surgery, Mayo Clinic College of Medicine, Mayo Clinic, Rochester, Minnesota

MELISSA M. ERICKSON, MD
Orthopedic Spine Fellow, Mayo Clinic College of Medicine, Mayo Clinic, Rochester, Minnesota

LACEY A. FELDMAN, BA
Clinical Research Coordinator, Tower Orthopaedics and Neurosurgical Spine Institute, Beverly Hills, California

BEN J. GARRIDO, MD
Founding Member, Lake Norman Orthopedic Spine Center, Mooresville, North Columbia

DAVID GENDELBERG, BS
Research Fellow, Department of Orthopaedic Surgery, Rothman Institute, Thomas Jefferson University and Hospitals, Philadelphia, Pennsylvania

ZIYA L. GOKASLAN, MD
Department of Neurosurgery, Johns Hopkins University, Baltimore, Maryland

GREGORY GRABOWSKI, MD
Assistant Professor, Department of Orthopaedics and Sports Medicine, University of South Carolina School of Medicine, Columbia, South Carolina

CHAMBLISS HARROD, MD
Spine Surgery Fellow, Department of
Orthopaedic Surgery, Thomas Jefferson
University and Hospitals, The Rothman
Institute, Philadelphia, Pennsylvania

MELVIN D. HELGESON, MD
Spine Fellow, Department of Orthopaedic
Surgery, Rothman Institute, Thomas Jefferson
University and Hospitals, Philadelphia,
Pennsylvania

ALAN S. HILIBRAND, MD
Professor, Department of Orthopaedic
Surgery, Thomas Jefferson University and The
Rothman Institute, Philadelphia, Pennsylvania

MARK E. JACOBSON, MD
Resident Physician, Department of
Orthopaedics, The Ohio State University,
Columbus, Ohio

JAMES D. KANG, MD
Professor of Orthopaedic and Neurological
Surgery, Department of Orthopaedic Surgery,
University of Pittsburgh, Pittsburgh,
Pennsylvania

CHRISTOPHER K. KEPLER, MD, MBA
Spine Fellow, Department of Orthopaedic
Surgery, Thomas Jefferson University and The
Rothman Institute, Philadelphia, Pennsylvania

SAFDAR N. KHAN, MD
Assistant Professor, Department of
Orthopaedics, The Ohio State University,
Columbus, Ohio

CARL LAURYSSEN, MD
Tower Orthopaedics and Neurosurgical Spine
Institute, Beverly Hills, California

BRANDON D. LAWRENCE, MD
Assistant Professor, Department of
Orthopaedics, University of Utah, Salt Lake
City, Utah

PAUL C. MCAFEE, MD, MBA
The Spine and Scoliosis Center, St. Joseph's
Hospital, Baltimore; Chief of Spinal Surgery,
Orthopaedic Associates of Towson, Towson,
Maryland

MARK M. MIKHAEL, MD
Spine Surgery Fellow, Department of
Orthopaedic Surgery, UCLA Comprehensive
Spine Center, Santa Monica, California

CAMILO A. MOLINA, BA
Department of Neurosurgery, Johns Hopkins
University, Baltimore, Maryland

SERGEY NECKRYSH, MD
Assistant Professor, Department of
Neurosurgery, University of Illinois, Chicago,
Illinois

PABLO R. PAZMIÑO, MD
SpineCal, Santa Monica, California

MIGUEL A. PELTON, BS
Research Assistant, Department of Orthopedic
Surgery, Rush University Medical Center,
Chicago, Illinois

JEFFREY A. RIHN, MD
Assistant Professor, Department of
Orthopaedic Surgery, Thomas Jefferson
University and Hospitals, The Rothman
Institute, Philadelphia, Pennsylvania

RICK C. SASSO, MD
Clinical Associate Professor and Chief of Spine
Surgery, Indiana University School of
Medicine, Department of Orthopaedic Surgery,
Indiana Spine Group, Indianapolis, Indiana

BEHNAM SALARI, DO, MS
The Spine and Scoliosis Center, St. Joseph's
Hospital, Baltimore; Maryland Spinal
Reconstructive Surgery Fellowship, Towson,
Maryland

JOSEPH SCHWARTZ, BS
Medical Student, Rush University Medical
Center School of Medicine, Chicago, Illinois

DANIEL M. SCIUBBA, MD
Department of Neurosurgery, Johns Hopkins
University, Baltimore, Maryland

GURSUKHMAN S. SIDHU, MBBS
Research Fellow, Department of Orthopaedic
Surgery, The Rothman Institute, Thomas
Jefferson University and Hospitals,
Philadelphia, Pennsylvania

KRZYSZTOF B. SIEMIONOW, MD
Assistant Professor, Department of
Orthopaedic Surgery, University of Illinois,
Chicago, Illinois

KERN SINGH, MD
Assistant Professor, Department of Orthopedic
Surgery, Rush University Medical Center,
Chicago, Illinois

ALEXANDER R. VACCARO, MD, PhD
Professor and Vice Chairman, Department of
Orthopaedic Surgery, The Rothman Institute,
Thomas Jefferson University and Hospitals,
Philadelphia, Pennsylvania

JEFFREY C. WANG, MD
Professor of Orthopaedic Surgery and
Neurosurgery, Department of Orthopaedic
Surgery, UCLA Comprehensive Spine Center,
Santa Monica, California

CHRISTOPHER F. WOLF, MD
Spine Surgery Fellow, Department of
Orthopaedic Surgery, UCLA Comprehensive
Spine Center, Santa Monica, California

Contents

The evolution of occipitocervical fixation and new rigid universal screw-rod construct technology has allowed secure anchorage at each level of the occipitocervical junction with the elimination of rigid external orthoses. Rigid occipitocervical instrumentation constructs have achieved higher fusion rates and less postoperative immobilization-associated complications. Outcomes have improved compared with former nonrigid instrumentation techniques; however, with advances of rigid occipitocervical stabilization capability have come new challenges, risks, and operative techniques. A thorough understanding of the relevant cervical bony and soft tissue anatomy is essential for safe implantation and a successful outcome.

The atlantoaxial motion segment, which is responsible for half of the rotational motion in the cervical spine, is a complex junction of the first (C1) and second (C2) cervical vertebrae. Destabilization of this joint is multifactorial and can lead to pathologic motion with neurologic sequelae. Posterior spinal fixation of the C1-C2 articulation in the presence of instability has been well described in the literature. Early reports of interspinous/interlaminar wiring have evolved into modern-day pedicle screw/translaminar constructs, with excellent results. The success of a C1-C2 posterior fusion rests on appropriate indications and surgical techniques.

The subaxial and cervicothoracic junction is a relatively difficult area for spine surgeons to navigate. Because of different transitional stressors at the junction of the smaller cervical vertebrae and the larger thoracic segments, proximity to neurovascular structures, and complex anatomy, extreme care and precision must be assumed during fixation in these regions. Lateral mass screws, pedicle screws, and translaminar screws are currently the standard of choice in the subaxial cervical and upper thoracic spine. This article addresses the relevant surgical anatomy, pitfalls, and pearls associated with each of these fixation techniques.

This article details the controversies associated with the different treatment strategies in patients with cervical spondylotic myelopathy. The natural history, incidence, pathophysiology, physical examination, and imaging findings are discussed followed by the indications, techniques, and outcomes of patients treated with posterior cervical decompression via decompressive laminectomy, laminectomy and instrumented fusion, and laminoplasty.

Cervical spondylotic myelopathy (CSM) is a slowly progressive disease resulting from age-related degenerative changes in the spine that can lead to spinal cord dysfunction and significant functional disability. The degenerative changes and abnormal motion lead to vertebral body subluxation, osteophyte formation, ligamentum flavum hypertrophy, and spinal canal narrowing. Repetitive movement during normal cervical motion may result in microtrauma to the spinal cord. Disease extent and location dictate the choice of surgical approach. Anterior spinal decompression and instrumented fusion is successful in preventing CSM progression and has been shown to result in functional improvement in most patients.

Adjacent segment disease (ASD) was described after long-term follow-up of patients treated with cervical fusion. The term describes new-onset radiculopathy or myelopathy referable to a motion segment adjacent to previous arthrodesis and often attributed to alterations in the biomechanical environment after fusion. Evidence suggests that ASD affects between 2% and 3% of patients per year. Although prevention of ASD was one major impetus behind the development of motion-sparing surgery, the literature does not yet clearly distinguish a difference in the rate of ASD between fusion and disk replacement. Surgical techniques during index surgery may reduce the rate of ASD.

Vertebral artery and esophageal injuries are rare but feared complications of cervical spine surgery. Appropriate understanding of treatment algorithms for prompt intervention in the event of a vertebral artery injury minimizes the risk of exsanguination and/or profound neurologic consequences. Esophageal injuries are often more subtle, and although intraoperative injuries can sometimes be diagnosed at the time of surgery, they frequently do not present until the week after surgery. They can additionally be seen as a late complication of instrumentation usage and/or failure. Expedient diagnosis and management of these injuries minimize their impact and allow for optimal treatment outcome.

The bony spine is overall the third most common site for distant cancer metastasis, with the cervical spine involved in approximately 8 to 20% of metastatic spine disease cases. Diagnosis and management of metastatic spine disease requires disease categorization into the compartment involved, pathology of the lesion, and anatomic region involved. The diagnostic approach should commence with careful physical examination, and the workup should include plain radiographs, magnetic resonance imaging, computed tomography, and bone scintigraphy. Management ranges from palliative nonoperative to aggressive surgical treatment. Optimal management requires proper patient selection to individualize the most appropriate treatment modality.

explained to the patient during the informed consent process. This article provides the spine care provider with an understanding of how to appropriately evaluate and manage the most common cervical conditions that require revision cervical spine surgery.

Minimally invasive approaches and operative techniques are becoming increasingly popular for the treatment of cervical spine disorders. Minimally invasive spine surgery attempts to decrease iatrogenic muscle injury, decrease pain, and speed postoperative recovery with the use of smaller incisions and specialized instruments. This article explains in detail minimally invasive approaches to the posterior spine, the techniques for posterior cervical foraminotomy and arthrodesis via lateral mass screw placement, and anterior cervical foraminotomy. Complications are also discussed. Additionally, illustrated cases are presented detailing the use of minimally invasive surgical techniques.

Orthopedic Clinics of North America

THE CLINICS ARE NOW AVAILABLE ONLINE!

Access your subscription at:
www.theclinics.com

Orthopedic Clinics of North America

Preface

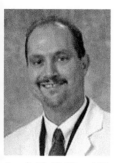 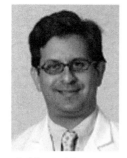

Frank M. Phillips, MD   Safdar N. Khan, MD
Guest Editors

It has been an incredible honor to serve as guest editors of the January 2012 edition of the *Orthopedic Clinics of North America* titled "Treatment of Complex Cervical Spine Disorders." This has, no doubt, been a labor of love and we have had the great fortune of collaborating with multiple thought leaders in the field of cervical spine surgery. As our understanding of the etiology and pathogenesis of complex cervical disorders has improved, so has the stringency of evaluation of surgical treatment of these conditions. Modern diagnostic evaluations coupled with evidence-based algorithms have changed the way we approach patients with these challenging conditions and we hope that the articles contained within this issue will educate and inspire members of the orthopedic community who take care of these patients.

This issue is a compendium of evidence-based articles pertaining to complex cervical disorders written by some of the world leaders in the field of spine surgery. This is our opportunity to formally thank each and every contributor; we approached their busy timelines with a request for "one more article" and each and every one of the authors stood up to the challenge. They have contributed collectively to an absolutely outstanding body of work. The greatest strength contained within these pages is the collective years of experience and wisdom from each author translated into clinical case scenarios: "The eye sees what the mind knows" and each contributor to this issue has provided cases that are controversial and challenging at best.

We would like to extend our sincerest gratitude to the journal's previous managing editor, Deb Dellapena, for her support of this issue. Furthermore, we are in tremendous debt of the current managing editor, David Parsons, and his entire staff for all of their time and patience devoted to this issue. Our thanks and gratitude extend to our families for their support. Finally, we urge the reader to appreciate that the strength of this issue is in the collective brilliance of the contributors and any deficiencies contained herein are exclusively ours.

Sincerely,

Frank M. Phillips, MD
Rush University Medical Center
1611 West Harrison Street, Suite 300
Chicago, IL 60612, USA

Safdar N. Khan, MD
Department of Orthopaedics
The Ohio State University
4110 Cramblett Hall
Columbus, OH 43210, USA

E-mail addresses:
fphillips@rushortho.com (F.M. Phillips)
safdar.khan@osumc.edu (S.N. Khan)

doi:10.1016/j.ocl.2011.10.002
0030-5898/12/$ – see front matter

orthopedic.theclinics.com

Occipitocervical Fusion

Ben J. Garrido, MD[a], Rick C. Sasso, MD[b],*

KEYWORDS

• Occipitocervical fusion • Fixation • Screw • Immobilization

---

Key Points

1. Preoperative imaging studies must be thoroughly reviewed for vertebral artery aberrant paths or inadequate bone stock for safe screw placement.

2. Meticulous attention to dissection is required to avoid excessive C1-2 venous sinusoid bleeding and to appreciate bony anatomic landmarks for safe instrumentation.

3. Planning and thorough familiarity with upper cervical spine anatomy are critical.

4. Versatile fixation techniques should be familiar and applied if bony anatomy precludes use of C2 pedicle screw instrumentation.

5. Appropriate patient positioning and visualization with intraoperative fluoroscopy are needed to facilitate both exposure and instrumentation.

Occipitocervical fusion may be indicated for multiple disease processes that render the craniocervical junction unstable. The causes may include trauma, rheumatoid arthritis, infection, tumor, congenital deformity, and degenerative processes. This junctional area between the mobile cervical spne and the rigid cranium offers fixation challenges and has a high incidence of significant and devastating spinal cord injury. Historically, stabilization of this junction dates back to 1927 when Foerster[1] used a fibular strut graft construct. Since then, other nonrigid methods of stabilization have been trialed, including wire fixation, pin fixation, hook constructs, and many others with onlay bone graft and halo immobilization.[2] However, these options required cumbersome, prolonged, postoperative external immobilization, including a halo vest or Minerva jacket to improve fusion rates and sometimes extended bed rest with traction. In an attempt to improve fusion rates and clinical outcomes and reduce the use of external immobilization, rigid internal fixation evolved.

In the early 1990s occipitocervical plate and screw fixation was developed, which provided immediate rigidity to the spine, thus eliminating postoperative halo vest immobilization.[3–6] In addition, it was not necessary to pass a sublaminar wire, which was a risky aspect of the Luque fixation[7] technique. Despite these advantages, plate and screw constructs did have limitations. These included a fixed hole-to-hole distance that may not match patient anatomy, preventing optimal screw placement; plate bulk, limiting space for graft material; and an inability to compress or distract across interspaces.[8] Occipital plate fixation also limited the ability to place occipital screws along the midline, the thickest and strongest bone area in the occiput.

---

[a] Lake Norman Orthopedic Spine Center, Mooresville, NC, USA
[b] Department of Orhopaedic Surgery, Indiana University School of Medicine, Indiana Spine Group, Indianapolis, IN, USA
* Corresponding author.
E-mail address: rsasso@indianaspinegroup.com

Orthop Clin N Am 43 (2012) 1–9
doi:10.1016/j.ocl.2011.08.009

In the mid-1990s, with the advent of rod-screw instrumentation, the limitations of plates were eliminated. The screws provided excellent fixation, and the use of rods allowed unlimited screw placement. There was greater space for bone grafting, and the ability to compress or distract became available.[8]

Occipital fixation has also dramatically improved because of the use of rigid fixation with contoured rod-screw instrumentation. Bicortical placement in the thickest and strongest bone along the occipital midline offers a biomechanical advantage and promotes stability and rigidity and thereby increases fusion rates. A technique using offset connectors and rods has been described that optimizes the ability to place 6 occipital screws in the parasagittal plane along the midline.[9] Several studies have also compared the stability of various occipitocervical constructs[10–13] and demonstrated that rigid occipitocervical fixation is superior to wiring or other nonrigid techniques. A recent clinical comparison of short-term outcomes confirmed a statistically significant lower rate of complications and superior clinical outcomes with rigid versus nonrigid occipitocervical fusion constructs.[14]

With the development of universal screw-rod instrumentation, techniques for stable cervical screw anchors proliferated. C1 lateral mass screw fixation, C2 pedicle screw fixation, C2 translaminar screw fixation, C1-C2 transarticular screws, and subaxial lateral mass screws can now all attach either directly or through offset connectors to a longitudinal rod.[9] These common cervical anchors provide rigid stability and have been found to be biomechanically superior to previous nonrigid fusion constructs. Universal screw-rod internal instrumentation has improved fusion rates and allowed immediate stability. The evolution of this instrumentation technology has resulted in the best opportunity to improve clinical outcomes and mitigate complications associated with nonrigid constructs.

SURGICAL INDICATIONS

The occipitocervical junction is susceptible to a wide variety of pathologic conditions that predispose it to instability. Any patient with instability, as a result of trauma, rheumatoid arthritis, infection, and congenital or tumor causes, experiencing a neurologic deficit requires arthrodesis. All cases with traumatic dislocation require primary surgical stabilization with a posterior occiput to cervical fusion. Other causes include incompetent occipitocervical ligamentous structures or associated vertical migration of the odontoid with rheumatoid arthritis, although less common with the advent of antirheumatic medications.

ANATOMY

Stabilization of the occipitocervical junction requires comprehensive knowledge of the anatomy. For safe placement of occipital screws, anatomic knowledge of regional occipital bony thickness and location of venous sinuses is essential. Anatomic studies of the occiput have demonstrated that the external occipital protuberance is the thickest in the midline and decreases laterally to inferiorly.[15] Screw fixation is preferred below the level of the superior nuchal line to avoid a transverse sinus injury and along the dense midline ridge below the external occipital protruberance.[16] The superior sagittal sinus runs from the confluence of both transverse sinuses superiorly along the occipital midline (**Fig. 1**). The quality of this midline bone stock is optimal and is the ideal occiput screw fixation point desired.

For atlantoaxial instrumentation and fixation, multiple fixation methods may be used, including transarticular screws, C1 lateral mass screws, or C2 pedicle, pars, or translaminar screws. Transarticular screws require a drill trajectory that starts at the C7-T1 region. Thus, excessive kyphosis precludes the ability to obtain the approach angle. Likely, the presence of an irreducible C1-C2 subluxation, deficient C2 bony pars, or aberrant medialized vertebral artery excludes this option. These anatomic variations must be evaluated as part of the preoperative plan.

The atlas is a large ring composed of 2 large lateral masses connected by an anterior and posterior arch. The lateral masses are wedge shaped and are congruent with the occipital condyles. The posterior arch contains a groove

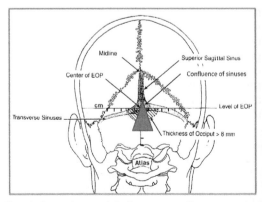

Fig. 1. Posterior occipital anatomy. Transverse and superior sagittal confluence of sinuses. Triangular area denotes ideal occipital screw placement. EOP, external occipital protuberance.

superiorly in which the vertebral artery lies. The C1 lateral mass lies anterior to the C1 posterior arch and must be carefully exposed to avoid venous plexus bleeding between C1 and C2. Subperiosteal reflection along the C1 posterior arch lateral undersurface facilitates lateral mass exposure without bleeding (**Fig. 2**). Once exposure of the posterior aspect of the C1 lateral mass is achieved, the C2 nerve with its venous sinusoid can be retracted caudally to expose the joint. Width of the C1 lateral mass should be established to avoid medial or lateral screw placement and potential spinal cord or vertebral artery injury, respectively. After perimeter margins are delineated, C1 lateral mass screw may be placed as popularized by Harms and Melcher.[13]

The axis is unique with the dens projecting cranially from the body to articulate with the anterior arch of the atlas and transverse ligament. Large lateral masses project laterally from the body. The lateral masses connect to the posterior elements through pedicles and a narrow bony isthmus or pars interarticularis. The C2 spinous process is bifid and serves as an attachment of the nuchal ligaments and cranial rotator muscles. The course of the vertebral arteries through the axis is variable and must be understood to minimize injury during surgery (**Fig. 3**). There are several options for axis screw fixation dependent on patient anatomy and surgeon preference. C2 pedicles should be evaluated on computed tomographic images for bony deficiency or a high-riding vertebral artery that would exclude pedicle screw fixation as a viable option. It is mandatory to differentiate between a screw placed into the C2 pars interarticularis and one placed into the C2 pedicle. These screw sites are not identical and possess distinct challenges of insertion and different potential complications.

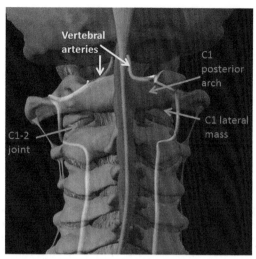

Fig. 3. Vertebral artery course through C1-2.

The confusion between the positions of these screw types lies in the unique anatomy of the C2 vertebra. The pars interarticularis is the region of bone between the superior and inferior articular processes. The pedicle is the region of bone that connects the posterior elements to the vertebral body. Because the superior articular process of C2 is extremely far anterior, the pars interarticularis is very large. This anterior position of the superior articular process also creates a very narrow and short window for connection to the C2 body, the pedicle.

The C2 pars interarticularis screw is in the exact position as a transarticular C1-C2 screw, except it stops short of the joint. The entry point is the same (approximately 3 mm superior and 3 mm lateral to the medial aspect of the C2-3 facet joint) (**Fig. 4**). As with transarticular C1-2 screws, the greatest risk associated with placement of the C2 pars screw is injury to the vertebral artery. Although this screw is a shorter version of the transarticular screw, it follows the same trajectory stopping short of the C1-2 joint.

The C2 pedicle screw follows the path of the pedicle into the vertebral body. For a screw to be inserted into the C2 vertebral body from the posterior elements, it by definition has to pass through the pedicle. The entry point is significantly cephalad to the entrance for the pars screw and slightly lateral (see **Fig. 4**). The medial angulation is significantly more than that of the pars screw, approximately 20° to 30°, although the pars screw is placed almost straight ahead. This cephalad starting point and medial angulation makes the pedicle screw less likely to injure the vertebral artery. The artery runs from medial to lateral in front of the C2-3 facet joint. The pedicle screw starts cephalad

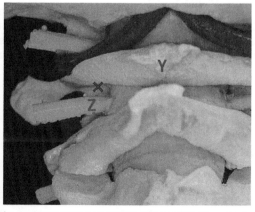

Fig. 2. Bony anatomy: C1 lateral mass (X), C1 posterior arch proper (Y), C1-2 joint below the C2 nerve root (Z).

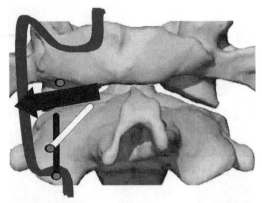

Fig. 4. Screw entry points for C1, C2, and pars versus pedicle screw fixation and their relationship to the vertebral artery and C2 nerve root. The starting points and trajectory for C2 pars (*purple*) and pedicle (*white*) screws are shown. The vertebral artery is red. The blue arrow is the C2 nerve root. The gray dot above the arrow is the starting point for the C1 lateral screw mass.

from the artery compared with the pars screw where the artery may be medial or just anterior to the starting point (see **Fig. 4**). In addition, the pars screw does not have a steep medial trajectory and is closer to the artery as it moves toward the superior articular process. The C2 pedicle screw cephalad trajectory is also not as steep, approximately 30° compared with more than 45° with the pars screw, and can usually be placed through the incision. The pars and transarticular screws need to have a very steep cephalad trajectory to keep away from the vertebral artery, which usually requires placement through percutaneous stab incisions at the cervicothoracic junction.

SURGICAL TECHNIQUE

Initial evaluation of head position in relation to the chest is important and can determine a potential dislocation and its direction. Anterior, posterior, or vertical displacement injuries can occur and require reduction. Although tong traction can play a role in reducing deformities or dislocations,

it has potential for harm if not used judiciously. For vertical displacement injuries, it is important not to further distract them with tong placement and perform expeditious definitive fixation. Anterior dislocations can be reduced via a roll under the shoulders, allowing the head to fall back. Likewise, posterior dislocations reduce simply by placing the head on a pillow or blankets, allowing it to translate forward. This reduction across the occipitocervical junction should occur under direct fluoroscopic visualization of the occiput and upper cervical spine. If surgical stabilization is delayed after any reduction, close and frequent evaluation, both clinically and radiographically, must be performed until definitive fixation. Patients with a cervical or occipitocervical injury can initially be placed in tong traction until operative fixation. No significant traction need be applied to this system; 4-7 kilograms suffice in maintaining a neutral anatomic position. Tong traction also denotes the severity of the injury to other health care personnel and offer a head handle for facilitating transfers and intraoperative head positioning.

Patients should be considered for an awake fiberoptic nasal or endotracheal intubation while neuromonitoring is performed. Patients will need spinal cord monitoring throughout the procedure. Prone positioning on the Jackson table using either a Mayfield 3-pin head holder or Gardner-Wells tong axial traction with Mayfield headrest is our preferred method. After the patient is positioned, radiographic studies are performed to confirm satisfactory anatomic alignment.

The posterior cervical approach is facilitated with slight cervical kyphotic positioning and minimal traction. It is critical to correct sagittal alignment before fusion. The patient is also placed in a reverse Trendelenburg position to decrease venous bleeding (**Fig. 5**). Fusion can be done using a variety of fixation techniques; rod and screw fixation is our preference.

Rigid screw fixation is widely accepted for the occipitocervical junction and provides excellent stability and increases construct rigidity.[8–10] We place our cervical fixation in the form of C2 laminar

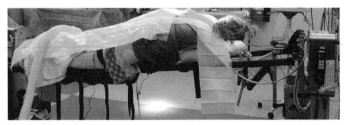

Fig. 5. Intraoperative patient positioning: prone position, reverse Trendelenburg, and Mayfield headrest. Although an option, no axial traction was used in this example.

or pedicle screws with C1 lateral mass screws. Posterior C1 arch lateral exposure should not extend beyond 15 mm from midline on the cephalad aspect; any further dissection could result in vertebral artery injury (see **Fig. 4**). Dissection to the lateral mass of C1 at the C1-2 joint requires a significant anterior course from the lateral posterior C1 arch (see **Fig. 2**). During this exposure, an extensive venous plexus surrounding the C2 nerve root can be a significant source of bleeding. Subperiosteal dissection to this anterior C1 lateral mass is critical to mobilize the C2 nerve and its venous plexus. The screw entry point is at the cephalad, center aspect of the lateral mass, and exposure is facilitated by caudal C2 nerve root displacement (see **Fig. 2**). Lateral fluoroscopic images are then used to facilitate correct drill trajectory; medial angulation is usually 10° to 15°. It is important to note that the inferior rim of the C1 posterior arch may obstruct adequate visualization of the C1 lateral mass and appropriate drill trajectory. We recommend meticulously removing this inferior rim with a Kerrison rongeur or burr without cephalad penetration to avoid vertebral artery injury. This removal improves drill and screw placement angle.

When placing a C2 pedicle screw, the trajectory has a greater medial angulation compared with a C1 lateral mass screw. Approximately 20° to 30° of medial angulation is required for placing a C2 pedicle screw. The medial border of the pedicle is palpated with a penfield to help guide the trajectory and avoid medial cortical breach and neurologic injury. Excessive lateral placement can also result in injuring the vertebral artery through violation of the transverse foramen. Lateral fluoroscopic imaging can also help guide the approximate 25° cephalad trajectory. We recommend removing any parallax on intraoperative fluoroscopic views to ensure perfect screw superimposition. Our preference is to use 3.5-mm screws with a length range of 22 to 30 mm. If preoperative studies demonstrate insufficient pedicle bone stock, other fixation options must be considered. Translaminar screws may be a viable option if safe placement of C2 pedicle screws is not possible. Screws are placed into the C2 lamina using a crossed trajectory with contralateral starting points on the spinolaminar junction. The junction width must be evaluated for placement of 2 screws without compromising or fracturing the spinous process. The surgeon must dock at the spinolaminar junction and target contralateral facet in line with the lamina. A pilot hole must be created with starting awl, leaving enough room for the contralateral translaminar screw along the width of the spinolaminar junction.

The first screw is positioned at the cephalad, superior aspect of the spinolaminar confluence, and the contralateral screw caudal and inferior to it in line with the lamina. We would caution from starting high on the spinous process to avoid a fracture. Using a small drill bit, the surgeon must drill under power through to the contralateral lamina using tactile feel throughout the anatomic bony trajectory, taking care to stay within lamina and avoid breaching ventrally into canal. The surgeon must then measure for screw length off calibrated drill and place screws manually to avoid overtightening or fracturing the spinous process. The final intraoperative fluoroscopic images must be obtained to confirm all cervical screw positions.

Once the cervical spine anchors are in place, our preferred occipital fixation includes placement of 3 paired screws just off midline in the parasagittal plane. Rods are bent to the appropriate occipitocervical sagittal lordotic angle, contoured to lie flat on the occiput and cut so not to pass the superior nuchal line. Three medial offset connectors (**Fig. 6**), our preferred technique, are inserted on to the cephalad aspect of each rod, and the best zone for occiput screw insertion is defined. The most cephalad screws are placed immediately lateral to the external occipital protuberance below the superior nuchal line and close to midline. Subsequent caudal screws are placed as close to midline as possible to maximize bone purchase (**Fig. 7**). Screws should not be placed inferior to the inferior nuchal line where the bone is thin. Bicortical occipital fixation is attained for both stronger purchase and avoidance of screw abutment against the far cortex and risk of stripping proximal cortical threads. During hole preparation, if a cerebrospinal fluid leak or venous

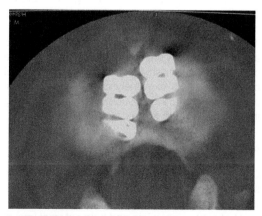

Fig. 6. Medial offset connectors link midline occiput screws to occipitocervical rods bent to the anatomic sagittal angle.

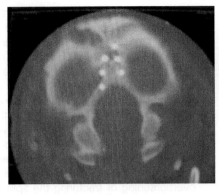 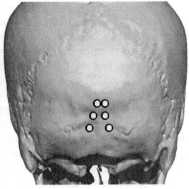

Fig. 7. Midline occipital screw fixation points.

bleeding develops, quick placement of the screw will suffice. On completion, a total of 6 occipital bicortical paramedian fixation points are established with an average screw length of 10 mm. After occipital and cervical screws are placed, a rod is bent to match a neutral sagittal occipitocervical angle, contoured to lie flat on the occiput and cut to not pass the superior nuchal line. Attention to head position for fusion should avoid extension, flexion, or rotation and requires a neutral occipitocervical angle. With the contoured rod sagittal apex about the posterior arch of the atlas, the cephalad aspect of the rod can easily be rotated toward the midline. Rod rotational variability and offset connectors provide great coronal plane versatility optimizing connection to the occiput. The rod is then connected to cervical fixation points directly or with offset connectors if required.

An optimal environment for fusion is prepared by decortication using a high speed burr, and bone graft is placed underneath and lateral to the rod construct. Many options exist for bone graft; however, autograft remains the gold standard in most cervical fusions despite associated morbidity of harvest sites including the iliac crest. If decompression is performed, it is important to avoid graft placement into the defect and on the dura. With rigid internal fixation, occipitocervical pseudarthrosis is extremely rare even with local bone graft and graft extenders. Thus, harvesting iliac crest autograft is becoming less common.

POTENTIAL COMPLICATIONS

Complications of occipitocervical fusion can be serious. Many of the early adverse events were associated with nonrigid fixation, including placement of sublaminar wires and halo external immobilization required afterward. Complications with sublaminar wire placement, including loss of

fixation, acute or chronic spinal cord and brain stem injury, and associated halo immobilization problems including pin tract infections, osteomyelitis, nerve injury, pulmonary complications, and death, have been described.[2,8,14] Nonrigid fixation lacks rotational stability and has been shown to have higher complication rates compared with rigid fixation.[14] Biomechanical studies have also shown superior stability with rigid screw fixation.[10–12]

Occipital screw misplacement can also lead to problems. If not positioned close to the superior nuchal line, then inadequate occipital thickness may be encountered and poor purchase may result. Also, if the far cortex of the occipital bone is not drilled or tapped, the screw can strip its proximal cortex threads when it reaches the far cortex. If a significant amount of occipital bone has been resected or lost, placing 3 screws below the superior nuchal line may be very difficult. If screws are then applied cephalad to the superior nuchal line, the transverse venous sinus may be encountered penetrating the intracranial venous sinus. An attempt to repair this sinus is problematic, and the best option is to simply place the screw.

Transarticular C1-2 screws require anatomic reduction intraoperatively to avoid complications of vertebral artery injury, neurologic deficit, or inadequate bony purchase. A precise drill trajectory is critical and is performed under biplanar fluoroscopic imaging or the use of a navigation system. These screws are potentially the most dangerous screw because of the potential for vertebral artery injury.[17,18] They may be contraindicated if anomalous vertebral artery anatomy exists; pronounced thoracic kyphosis inhibiting drill angle or proper C1-2 reduction is not feasible. This technique is technically demanding and has had variable vertebral artery injury rates reported

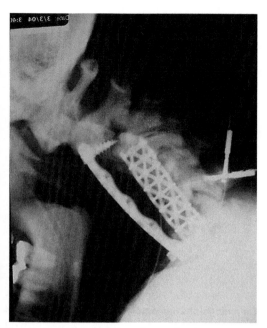

Fig. 8. Lateral cervical radiograph demonstrating previous anterior C3-6 corpectomy with cage/plate reconstruction.

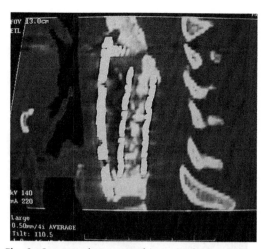

Fig. 9. Computed tomographic sagittal view demonstrating failure of a previous cervical corpectomy with kyphotic deformity.

in the literature. Wright and colleagues[17] have reported a 4% risk of injury. If vertebral artery injury does occur, the screw has to be placed across the joint and a postoperative angiogram is obtained. The surgeon should not drill across the contralateral joint if one vertebral artery is compromised.

C1 lateral mass screw placement can also result in C2 nerve root injury and extensive venous plexus bleeding. Precise knowledge of the anatomy and entry point for the C1 lateral mass screw is required. Caution must be taken to avoid a medial starting point or medial penetration, which could result in dural or spinal cord injury. Bicortical fixation is not required and avoids potential injury to either the hypoglossal nerve or the internal carotid artery, which lie anterior to the C1 lateral mass.

C2 pedicle screws can also be a potential hazard to the vertebral artery if incorrect entry point is confused for that of the pars screw. C2 pedicle anatomic location must be clearly differentiated from the pars (see **Fig. 4**). The C2 pedicle entry point is more cephalad and lateral than the pars screw entry point. Most importantly, the greater medial trajectory of the C2 pedicle screw makes it less likely to injure the vertebral artery. Avoiding spinal cord injury through a medial cortical breech is also critical; hence the medial border of the pedicle is usually palpated to triangulate appropriate drill trajectory.

After instrumentation or decompression is performed, the optimal environment for fusion must be established. Autograft bone is the gold standard and should be placed into a bleeding decorticated cancellous bed. Decortication must be performed with a high-speed burr and graft placed underneath and lateral to the rod construct. If decompression is performed it is important to avoid graft placement into the defect and on the dura. Meticulous technique must be implemented when using the high-speed burr over an exposed spinal cord.

CASE

We illustrate the case of a 44-year-old woman who presented several months after a multilevel anterior cervical corpectomy and fusion performed at an outside facility. She complained of inability to use her hands and walk and cervical axial pain (**Fig. 8**). The patient was found to have an active infection with failure of hardware resulting in a kyphotic deformity (**Fig. 9**) on myelopathic examination findings. She was medically optimized, intravenous (IV) antibiotics were initiated, and posterior occipitocervical stabilization was performed (**Fig. 10**). The patient's myelopathy fully resolved, and the infection was treated with long term IV antibiotics without further need of an anterior debridement.

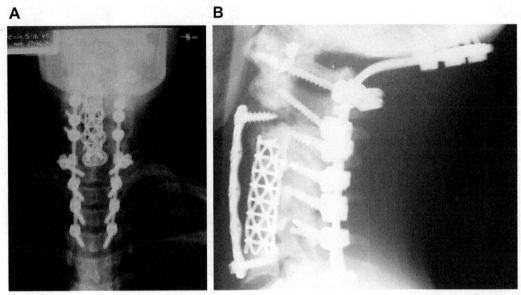

A   **B**

Fig. 10. (*A, B*) Postsurgical anteroposterior and lateral cervical radiographs demonstrating posterior occipitocervical fusion and correction of sagittal alignment.

SUMMARY

The evolution of occipitocervical fixation and new rigid universal screw-rod construct technology has allowed secure anchorage at each level of the occipitocervical junction with the elimination of rigid external orthoses. Rigid occipitocervical instrumentation constructs have achieved higher fusion rates and less postoperative immobilization-associated complications. Outcomes have improved compared with former nonrigid instrumentation techniques; however, with advances of rigid occipitocervical stabilization capability have come new challenges, risks, and operative techniques. A thorough understanding of the relevant cervical bony and soft tissue anatomy is essential for safe implantation and a successful outcome. Early ambulation is encouraged. A Miami J (Jerome Group Inc, Mount Laurel, NJ, USA) or Philadelphia collar (Charles Greiner & Co Inc, Westville, NJ, USA) can be used for 12 weeks postoperatively. These patients should be followed up closely for any progressive deformities or neurologic deficit that may develop after rigid occipitocervical fixation.

REFERENCES

1. Foerster O. Die leitungsbahmen des schmerzgefuhls und die chirurgischee behandlung der schmerzzustande. Berlin: Urbin and Schwarzenberg; 1927.
2. Vender JR, Rekito AJ, Harrison SJ, et al. The evolution of posterior cervical and occipitocervical fusion and instrumentation. Neurosurg Focus 2004;16:E9.
3. Lieberman IH, Webb JK. Occipito-cervical fusion using posterior titanium plates. Eur Spine J 1998;7: 349–65.
4. Sasso RC, Jeanneret B, Fischer K, et al. Occipitocervical fusion with posterior plate and screw instrumentation. A long-term follow up study. Spine 1994; 19:2364–8.
5. Smith MD, Anderson P, Grady MS. Occipitocervical arthrodesis using contoured plate fixation. An early report on a versatile fixation. Spine 1993;18: 1984–90.
6. Grob D, Dvorak J, Panjabi M, et al. The role of plate and screw fixation in occipitocervical fusion in rheumatoid arthritis. Spine 1994;19:2545–51.
7. Luque ER. The anatomic basis and development of segmental spinal instrumentation. Spine 1982;7: 256–9.
8. Stock GH, Vaccaro AR, Brown AK, et al. Contemporary posterior occipital fixation. J Bone Joint Surg Am 2006;88(7):1642–9.
9. Garrido BJ, Puschak TJ, Anderson PA, et al. Occipitocervical fusion using contoured rods and medial offset connectors. Description of a new technique. Orthopedics 2009;32(10):1–4.
10. Hurlbert RJ, Crawford NR, Choi WG, et al. A biomechanical evaluation of occipitocervical

instrumentation: screw compared with wire fixation. J Neurosurgery 1999;90(Suppl 1):84–90.

11. Oda I, Abumi K, Sell LC, et al. Biomechanical evaluation of five different occipito-atlanto-axial fixation techniques. Spine 1999;24:2377–82.

12. Sutterlin CE, Bianchi JR, Kunz DN, et al. Biomechanical evaluation of occipitocervical fixation devices. J Spinal Disord 2001;14:185–92.

13. Harms J, Melcher RP. Posterior C1-2 fusion with polyaxial screws and rod fixation. Spine 2001;26:2467–71.

14. Garrido BJ, Myo GK, Sasso RC. Rigid vs nonrigid occipitocervical fusion. A clinical comparison of short-term outcomes. J Spinal Disord 2011;24(1):20–3.

15. Roberts DA, Doherty BJ, Heggeness MH, et al. Quantitative anatomy of the occiput and the biomechanics of occipital screw fixation. Spine 1998;23:1100–7.

16. Zipnick RT, Merola AA, Gorup J, et al. Occipital morphology: an anatomic guide to internal fixation. Spine 1996;21:1719–24.

17. Wright NM, Lauryssen C. Vertebral artery injury in C1/C2 transarticular screw fixation: results of a survey of the AANS/CNS section on disorders of the spine and peripheral nerves. J Neurosurg 1998;88:634–40.

18. Sasso RC. Complications of posterior occipitocervical instrumentation. In: Vacarro AR, Regan JJ, Crawford AH, et al, editors. Complications of pediatric and adult spinal surgery. New York: Marcel Derker; 2004. p. 301–21.

C1-C2 Posterior Fixation: Indications, Technique, and Results

Mark E. Jacobson, MD[a], Safdar N. Khan, MD[a],*,
Howard S. An, MD[b]

KEYWORDS

- First cervical vertebra • Second cervical vertebra
- C1-C2 fixation • Spinal injury

The atlantoaxial motion segment is a complex junction of the first and second cervical vertebrae that is responsible for half of the rotational motion in the cervical spine. Destabilization of this joint is multifactorial and can lead to pathologic motion with neurologic sequelae. Static stability is conferred by both osseous and ligamentous contributions consisting primarily of the facet articulations, dens and fovea dentis, the facet capsule, and the transverse atlantal ligament. Dynamic stability arises from the multiple muscular attachments of the anterior arch and transverse process. Trauma, congenital malformation, inflammatory arthritides, and malignancy have all been implicated in the development of atlantoaxial instability. Since the first description of surgical treatment by Mixter and Osgood in 1910,[1] multiple techniques have been described to provide atlantoaxial stability in an effort to protect the space available for the spinal cord and prevent basilar invagination.

ANATOMIC CONSIDERATIONS

The first cervical vertebra (C1) consists of an anterior arch, a posterior arch, and two lateral masses, giving it a ringlike structure. The anterior tubercle on the anterior arch serves as an attachment site for the longus colli muscle; posteriorly, the fovea dentis serves as the articulation point for the

odontoid process of the second cervical vertebra (C2). The posterior arch provides a smooth edge for the attachment of the posterior atlanto-occipital membrane. The sulcus arteriae vertebralis is present behind each superior articular process and represents the superior vertebral notch. The vertebral artery and the first spinal nerve reside within this sulcus. The undersurface of the posterior arch provides an attachment surface for the posterior atlantoaxial ligament. The lateral masses of C1 have an inferior and a superior articular facet; the superior facet surface forms a cuplike articulating surface for the corresponding condyle of the occiput. The inferior articular facet surfaces articulate with C2 and permit rotation of the head. Anteriorly, at the level of the superior facet the important transverse atlantal ligament traverses the C1 ring, dividing the vertebral foramen into an anterior part, which contains the dens, and a posterior part, which encases the spinal cord. On occasion, the sulcus for the vertebral artery on the dorsal aspect of the atlas may be completely covered by an anomalous ossification, termed the ponticulus posticus.[2] The resulting foramen retains the vertebral artery and is referred to as the arcuate foramen.[3] Young and colleagues[2] retrospectively reviewed 464 lateral radiographs of the neck and determined a prevalence of 15.5% of the presence of

Disclosures: None.
[a] Department of Orthopaedics, The Ohio State University, 4110 Cramblett Hall, Columbus, OH 43210, USA
[b] Department of Orthopaedics, Rush University Medical Center, 1653 W. Congress Parkway, Chicago, IL 60612, USA
* Corresponding author.
E-mail address: safdar.khan@osumc.edu

Orthop Clin N Am 43 (2012) 11–18
doi:10.1016/j.ocl.2011.09.004

orthopedic.theclinics.com

this anomaly. The relevance of this finding is that some surgeons have advocated the starting point of a C1 lateral mass screw to be at the dorsal aspect of the posterior arch instead of the base of the lateral mass. The presence of an unidentified posticulus posticus may lead to iatrogenic injury to the vertebral artery.

The second cervical vertebra (C2) or axis forms a pivot by which the first vertebra rotates. The dens has an apex and neck at which it joins the body. An oval facet on its anterior surface allows articulation with the atlas. Posteriorly, neck of the dens is the insertion site of the transverse atlantal ligament. The apical odontoid ligament attaches along the apex, and caudally, along either side of the neck the alar ligaments attach, which connects the odontoid process to the occiput. The pedicles are covered by the superior articular surfaces that articulate with C1. The transverse processes are each perforated by the foramen transversarium via which the vertebral artery ascends at C6. After exiting the foramen of the axis, the artery courses laterally to pass through the foramen of the atlas. The vessel then courses posteromedially along the superior aspect of the atlas in the superior vertebral notch to enter the dura near the midline, before traveling through the foramen magnum to form the Circle of Willis. The left vertebral artery is dominant in 36% of patients, hypoplastic in 6%, and absent in 2%. The right is dominant in 23% of patients, hypoplastic in 9%, and absent in 3%. Equivalent right and left vertebral arteries are present in 41% of patients.[4]

Classic Indications

Trauma

In the setting of fracture, most surgeons determine atlantoaxial stability based on the integrity of the transverse atlantal ligament.[5] Jefferson fractures with combined lateral displacement of the C1 lateral masses on C2 of greater than 6.9 mm on an anterior-posterior radiograph of the odontoid process suggest that the transverse atlantal ligament has been torn.[6] Results of nonoperative management of displaced fractures have been poor.[7] There is controversy in the literature regarding appropriate surgical management.[5,8–10] Proposed treatments include halo brace immobilization, traction, atlantoaxial fusion, and more recently, C1 ring osteosynthesis.[5,6,8] Regardless of treatment method, postoperative radiographic assessment of stability is indicated.

Odontoid fractures represent 5% to 15% of all cervical spine injuries.[11] Anderson-D'alonzo Type II odontoid fractures are the most common odontoid injury, and result in atlantoaxial instability

requiring stabilization.[12] Although treatment of odontoid fractures remains controversial, atlantoaxial arthrodesis is an accepted treatment option.[11] In addition, placement of an odontoid screw in a morbidly obese patient or a patient with significant kyphosis may not be possible from an anterior approach, necessitating a posterior approach and atlantoaxial arthrodesis.[13]

Traumatic rupture of the transverse ligament without fracture is rare. In adult patients with intact atlantoaxial ligaments the anterior atlanto-dens interval is 3 mm with no change during flexion or extension.[6,14] Fielding and colleagues[15] demonstrated that "acute shift of the first on the second cervical vertebra under load does not exceed 3 millimeters if the transverse ligament is intact," and that following rupture the remaining structures are unable to stop further displacement. In this setting atlantoaxial fusion is indicated to protect the space available for the spinal cord.

Rheumatoid arthritis

Rheumatoid arthritis is a chronic autoimmune mediated inflammatory disorder characterized by synovial joint pannus formation and periarticular erosions. Following the hands and feet, the cervical spine is the most common site of involvement, often within 2 years of diagnosis.[16] Three types of instability are seen, usually in progression with advancement of disease: atlantoaxial subluxation, basilar invagination, and finally subaxial subluxation. The typical presentation is that of neck pain with positional temporal or suboccipatal radiation. Radiographic evidence of instability typically precedes neurologic symptoms. If the disease has progressed to basilar invagination or subaxial subluxation, extended fusion is indicated. Atlantoaxial arthrodesis is indicated in patients with intractable pain, progressive neurologic deficit, or myelopathy in patients with instability.[17] Some investigators have proposed surgery before the development of neurologic symptoms if the posterior atlanto-dens interval is less than 14 mm in the setting of atlantoaxial instability. Treatment prior to the development of myelopathy has been associated with improved outcomes.[16]

Congenital malformation

Os odontoideum represents an independent smoothly corticated ossicle of variable size, which is separated from the hypoplastic odontoid peg.[18] The etiology of os odontoideum remains controversial, with two distinct schools of thought. The congenital origin theory hypothesizes that the segmental anomaly present results from failure of fusion between the dens and the body of the axis.[19,20] The traumatic origin theory suggests that os odontoideum represents a late diagnosis of previously unrecognized odontoid type II fracture followed by avascular necrosis, nonunion, and ossicle remodeling.[18,21] Presentation may vary from an incidental finding, axial neck pain, or myelopathic deficits. In a recent review, Arvin and colleagues[18] suggest that "patients with unstable os odontoideum or those with a fixed deformity causing compression of the upper cervical/medullary junction should be offered surgery." Ventral or dorsal approach and fixation should be predicated on the direction of neurologic compression if present, as well as surgeon experience and comfort.

TECHNIQUE
Dorsal Wiring

History
The first surgical treatment of atlantoaxial instability was described by Mixter and Osgood[1] in 1910. These investigators reported using a braided silk suture looped around the posterior arch of the atlas under the spinous process of the axis as treatment for symptomatic atlantoaxial subluxation secondary to odontoid nonunion in a 15-year-old boy, with good results at 2-year follow-up. In 1939 Gallie[22] reported "recurrence of displacement can be guarded against by fastening the two vertebrae together by fine steel wire passed around the laminae or spines … and … bone grafts laid in the spines or on the laminae and articular facets."

Technique
The technique of modern dorsal wiring was described by Brooks and Jenkins[23] in 1978. After careful exposure of the spinous process and laminae of the axis and subperiosteal dissection of the posterior arch of the atlas, the opposing surfaces of the atlas and axis are prepared for bone graft. A suture is then placed on each side of the midline from proximal to distal under the arch of the atlas and subsequently under each laminae of the axis. The suture is then used as a guide to direct the looped end of two doubled 20-gauge stainless-steel wires. Two rectangular full-thickness autogenous iliac crest bone grafts are placed on either side of the midline in the prepared intralaminar space. The construct is secured by twisting the wires dorsally.

The technique of Brooks and Jenkins was modified by Dickman and colleagues[9] such that sublaminar wires need only be placed at a single level. Using this method a loop of #24 surgical steel is passed from distal to proximal under the posterior arch of the atlas. A single rectangular bicortical iliac crest bone graft with an inferior central notch is then placed over the spinous process of the axis dorsal to the free ends of surgical steel with the concavity opposed to the dura. The loop is then pulled caudally, where it is secured in a notch created on the inferior aspect of the C2 spinous process. One of the free ends of surgical steel is passed under the spinous process of the axis similarly to the loop, and compression is obtained by twisting the free ends 3 times per centimeter so that the graft, if trapped dorsal to the free wire, ends ventral to the loop. Postoperatively all patients were placed in halo immobilization for 3 months followed by a Philadelphia collar for 4 to 6 weeks.

Results
In their classic article Brooks and Jenkins[23] reported osseous fusion of the atlantoaxial joint in 93% of cases (13/14) who were available for follow-up. One patient died 8 weeks postoperatively of unknown cause. These results have been verified by several subsequent reports on fusion. Using the Sonntag modification of the Brooks fusion, Dickman and colleagues[9] reported osseous fusion in 89% of patients (31/35). Of note, a disproportionately high number (3/4) of these nonunions were treated for rheumatoid arthritis.

Complications and technical considerations
Complications of dorsal intralaminar and intraspinous wiring techniques were rare. Nonunion is a well-known complication of any arthrodesis procedure, and is discussed elsewhere in this article. Iatrogenic fracture of the posterior arch during wire tensioning necessitating extension of the fusion construct was reported by Brooks. Also concerning is the risk of dural tear or neurologic injury while passing sublaminar wires. This complication was not reported in the Brooks or Sonntag articles; however, other investigators have reported this at the axis.[24] Space available for the spinal cord decreases at more caudal levels, and the theoretical advantages of the Sonntag modification are worth considering. Although early reports of these techniques demonstrated excellent fusion results, more recent reports have suggested nonunion rates of up to 30%. Furthermore, the biomechanical superiority of the transarticular method is well documented.[25,26]

Transarticular Atlantoaxial Arthrodesis

Technique
Transarticular atlantoaxial fixation was first described by Magerl and Seemann[27] in 1987. In this technique the patient is positioned prone with the neck in neutral and the head in a tucked

position. A midline dorsal incision is created to expose the posterior elements of C1 to C3 with attention to the posterior aspect of the atlantoaxial facet joint. Before fixation, reduction of subluxation is performed with positioning or manual techniques such as the Halifax interlaminar clamp.[28] Through bilateral stab incisions a Kirschner wire is then directed down the C2 pedicle across the facet joint toward a point 3 to 4 mm posterior to the anterior tubercle of C1. A cannulated drill bit is then passed over the Kirschner wire, taking care not to inadvertently advance the wire. The pilot hole is then taped, and a solid 3.5-mm or cannulated 4.0 mm cortical screw is then placed bilaterally.[29] Use of a Herbert compression screw has also been described.[28] This construct is then supplemented with intralaminar iliac crest autograft and dorsal wiring using a dorsal wiring technique or interlaminar clamp.[28,29] Anomalous course of the vertebral artery, comminuted fracture, or other pathologic lesions made bilateral transarticular screw placement unsuitable in 7% to 17% of patients.[17,29–31] Given the added stability of instrumentation, halo immobilization is usually avoided except in the instance of severe osteoporosis.[17,28–30]

Results
Reports have documented osseous fusion in 96% to 99% of cases using this technique.[17,29,30,32] Improvement of neck pain, anterior atlanto-dens interval, and neurologic symptoms were findings at long-term clinical follow-up in the majority of cases.[17,28,30,31]

Complications and technical considerations
While the definition of screw malposition is variable in the literature, the reported incidence is 2% to 15%.[30,32,33] Fortunately, the incidence of vertebral artery injury is low (2.4%), with several large series reporting no vertebral artery

injury.[29,30,32,33] Although the safety of the procedure has been well documented, the complex anatomy at the atlantoaxial junction and technical demands of the surgical procedure should not be underestimated. Apfelbaum[34] reported one instance of bilateral vertebral artery injury resulting in death in a series of 40 patients, Marcotte and colleagues[35] reported two cases of dural tears in a series of 18 patients, and Coric and colleagues[36] reported transarticular screw-induced arteriovenous fistula. Preoperative imaging is paramount in detecting an anomalous vertebral artery course that would preclude screw placement. Paramore and colleagues[37] assessed a series of computed tomography (CT) scans for determining the safety of potential screw trajectory, and concluded that 18% to 23% of patients "may not be suitable for posterior C1-2 transarticular screw fixation on at least one side." Complete reduction of atlantoaxial subluxation and appropriate monitoring during screw insertion further reduce the risk of inadequate screw placement.[33] When bilateral fixation is not possible, Song and colleagues[31] demonstrated that adequate stability could be achieved using a unilateral transarticular screw with 100% osseous union in 19 cases.

Polyaxial Screw and Rod Fixation

Technique
In 2001 Harms and Melcher[38] described a novel posterior fixation method that minimized the risk of injury to the vertebral artery, and allowed intraoperative reduction and fixation of the atlantoaxial complex. A dorsal approach is used with subperiosteal dissection from the occiput to C3-C4. Exposure of the C1-C2 joint with particular attention to the superior surface of the C2 pars interarticularis is critical for placement of the C1 lateral mass screw. The C2 dorsal root ganglion is retracted caudally and straight or slightly convergent

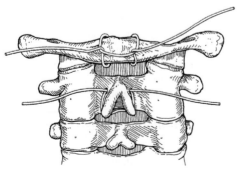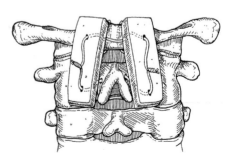

Fig. 1. The authors' preferred interspinous wiring technique for C1-C2 posterior fusions. (*Adapted from* Grob D, An HS. Posterior occiput and C1-C2 instrumentation. In: An HS, Cotler JM, editors. Spinal instrumentation. 2nd edition. Philadelphia: Lippincott Williams and Wilkins; 1999. p. 198.)

3.5 mm C1 lateral mass screws are placed from an entry point at the middle of the junction of the C1 posterior arch and the midpoint of the posterior inferior aspect of the C1 lateral mass.[38] C2 pedicle screws are placed from an entry point in the cranial and medial quadrant of the isthmus surface of C2 directed 20° to 30° in a convergent and cephalad direction predetermined by preoperative imaging.[38] The C1 lateral mass screw is left proud to allow rotation of the polyaxial screw head and to prevent C2 nerve root irritation. Reduction of subluxation can be achieved under direct fluoroscopic guidance by positional techniques or manipulation of the instrumentation. Whereas Harms and Melcher[38] recommended posterior C1 and C2 decortication and autogenous bone grafting for osseous fusion, Ni and colleagues[39] suggested a modification such that bicortical iliac crest graft is compressed between the posterior arch of C1 and the lamina of C2 using the rod and screw construct for graft compression. The authors' preferred fusion technique is to use a modified Gallie wiring with compression of corticocancellous allograft (**Fig. 1**). The pedicle/lateral mass screw construct provides stability; however, the authors believe that fusion is afforded by wiring/corticocancellous compression grafting.

Results

Osseous fusion at 3 to 6 months of follow-up is reported as from 94% to 100% using the polyaxial screw and rod technique.[38–40] A statistically significant improvement in postoperative neurologic status and subjectively reported neck has been reported.[39]

Complications

Screw malposition has varied from 0% to 4% in the atlas and 0% to 7% in the axis.[38–40] Four of the 28 patients presented by Stulik and colleagues[40] suffered from paresthesias in the region innervated by the greater occipital nerve, with all but one eventually resolving. Terterov and colleagues[41] reported symptomatic compression of the vertebral artery by the rod of a Harms-type construct. There are two reports of proximal rod migration through the base of the skull in the setting of atlantoaxial nonunion following the Harms technique.[42,43]

The risk of injury to the vertebral artery during placement of screws for atlantoaxial fixation is highly associated with screw malpositioning. Unidentified anomalous course of the vertebral artery increases this risk. There have been reports of erosion on the C2 lateral mass and pars by the artery itself, and asymmetric grooving of the C2 pars. In a study by Abou Madawi and colleagues,[44] 52% of their cadaveric specimens had an asymmetric course. Igarashi and colleagues[45] reported that the differences of the pars width on the superior surface of C2 averaged 1.2 ± 0.9 mm, the pars width on the inferior

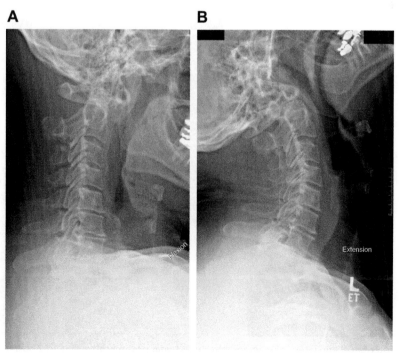

A   **B**

Fig. 2. Flexion (*A*) and extension (*B*) views of patient showing os odontoideum with marked instability at C1-C2.

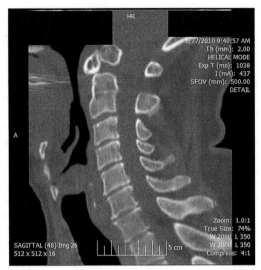

Fig. 3. Computed tomography scan revealing os odontoideum.

surface averaged 1.0 ± 0.8 mm, and the pars height averaged 1.2 ± 1.0 mm.

C2 Translaminar Constructs

Leonard and Wright[46] described a new technique for rigid screw fixation of the axis involving the insertion of polyaxial screws into the laminae of C2 in a bilateral, crossing fashion; they then incorporated these fixation points into atlantoaxial fixation or subaxial cervical constructs. This technique allows safer rigid fixation of C2, as the screws are not inserted near the vertebral artery. The caveat, however, is that unlike the transarticular or C1-C2 lateral mass/pedicles screw techniques of atlantoaxial fixation, this technique requires intact posterior elements of C2.

Technique
Patients are placed in the prone position with the head maintained in the neutral position using a head holder. The posterior arch of C1 is identified and the lateral masses are appropriately visualized. The spinous process, laminae, and medial lateral masses of C2 are then meticulously exposed. C1 lateral mass screws are placed using the Harms technique already described. The high-speed drill is used to open a small unicortical window at the C2 spinolaminar junction. Using a hand drill, the contralateral lamina is carefully drilled to a depth of 30 mm, with the drill angulated to match the contralateral laminar surface. A small ball-tipped probe is used to palpate the length of the drill hole to verify that no cortical breach into the spinal canal has occurred. A 30 mm polyaxial screw is carefully inserted along the same trajectory as the drill hole. The screw head thus sits at the spinolaminar junction on the right, with the

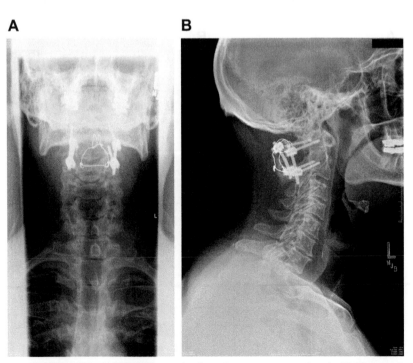

Fig. 4. Anteroposterior (*A*) and lateral (*B*) radiographs show 1-year postoperative s/p C1-C2 posterior spinal fusion with C1 lateral mass screws and C2 pedicle screws, with modified Gallie interspinous wiring.

length of the screw threads within the left lamina. Using the same technique a 30 mm screw is placed into the right lamina. After screw placement, all exposed laminar surfaces are decorticated and prepared for bone graft. The C1 lateral mass screws are connected to the C2 laminar screws with posterior rods.

Case example

The patient is a 55-year-old man who had a long-standing history of right-sided radicular pain with axial neck pain. Plain radiographs revealed an os odontoideum and flexion-extension radiographs revealed evidence of instability of the C1-C2 articulation (**Fig. 2**). CT scans revealed foraminal narrowing at C3-C4, C4-C5, and C5-C6. He underwent a C1-C2 posterior spinal fusion with modified Gallie wiring with structural allograft and right-sided foraminotomy of C3 to C6 (**Fig. 3**). The patient tolerated the procedure well, and returned to follow-up (**Fig. 4**) at 1 year with all symptoms completely resolved.

SUMMARY

Posterior spinal fixation of the C1-C2 articulation in the presence of instability has been well described in the literature. Early reports of interspinous/interlaminar wiring have evolved into modern-day pedicle screw/translaminar constructs, with excellent results. The success of a C1-C2 posterior fusion rests on appropriate indications and surgical techniques.

REFERENCES

1. Mixter SJ, Osgood RB. IV. Traumatic lesions of the atlas and axis. Ann Surg 1910;51(2):193–207.
2. Young JP, Young PH, Ackermann MJ, et al. The ponticulus posticus: implications for screw insertion into the first cervical lateral mass. J Bone Joint Surg Am 2005;87(11):2495–8.
3. Hasan M, Shukla S, Siddiqui MS, et al. Posterolateral tunnels and ponticuli in human atlas vertebrae. J Anat 2001;199(Pt 3):339–43.
4. Tokuda K, Miyasaka K, Abe H, et al. Anomalous atlantoaxial portions of vertebral and posterior inferior cerebellar arteries. Neuroradiology 1985;27(5):410–3.
5. Koller H, Resch H, Tauber M, et al. A biomechanical rationale for C1-ring osteosynthesis as treatment for displaced Jefferson burst fractures with incompetency of the transverse atlantal ligament. Eur Spine J 2010;19(8):1288–98.
6. Spence KF Jr, Decker S, Sell KW. Bursting atlantal fracture associated with rupture of the transverse ligament. J Bone Joint Surg Am 1970;52(3):543–9.
7. Dvorak MF, Johnson MG, Boyd M, et al. Long-term health-related quality of life outcomes following Jefferson-type burst fractures of the atlas. J Neurosurg Spine 2005;2(4):411–7.
8. Levine AM, Edwards CC. Fractures of the atlas. J Bone Joint Surg Am 1991;73(5):680–91.
9. Dickman CA, Sonntag VK, Papadopoulos SM, et al. The interspinous method of posterior atlantoaxial arthrodesis. J Neurosurg 1991;74(2):190–8.
10. Ruf M, Melcher R, Harms J. Transoral reduction and osteosynthesis C1 as a function-preserving option in the treatment of unstable Jefferson fractures. Spine (Phila Pa 1976) 2004;29(7):823–7.
11. Denaro V, Papalia R, Di Martino A, et al. The best surgical treatment for type II fractures of the dens is still controversial. Clin Orthop Relat Res 2011; 469(3):742–50.
12. Anderson LD, D'Alonzo RT. Fractures of the odontoid process of the axis. J Bone Joint Surg Am 1974;56(8):1663–74.
13. Menendez JA, Wright NM. Techniques of posterior C1-C2 stabilization. Neurosurgery 2007;60(1 Suppl 1): S103–11.
14. Grogono BJ. Injuries of the atlas and axis. J Bone Joint Surg Br 1954;36(3):397–410.
15. Fielding JW, Cochran GB, Lawsing JF 3rd, et al. Tears of the transverse ligament of the atlas. A clinical and biomechanical study. J Bone Joint Surg Am 1974;56(8):1683–91.
16. Kim DH, Hilibrand AS. Rheumatoid arthritis in the cervical spine. J Am Acad Orthop Surg 2005; 13(7):463–74.
17. Nagaria J, Kelleher MO, McEvoy L, et al. C1-C2 transarticular screw fixation for atlantoaxial instability due to rheumatoid arthritis: a seven-year analysis of outcome. Spine (Phila Pa 1976) 2009;34(26):2880–5.
18. Arvin B, Fournier-Gosselin MP, Fehlings MG. Os odontoideum: etiology and surgical management. Neurosurgery 2010;66(Suppl 3):22–31.
19. Currarino G. Segmentation defect in the midodontoid process and its possible relationship to the congenital type of os odontoideum. Pediatr Radiol 2002;32(1):34–40.
20. Flemming C, Hodson CJ. Os odontoideum; a congenital abnormality of the axis; case report. J Bone Joint Surg Br 1955;37(4):622–3.
21. Hawkins RJ, Fielding JW, Thompson WJ. Os odontoideum: congenital or acquired. A case report. J Bone Joint Surg Am 1976;58(3):413–4.
22. Gallie W. Fracture and dislocations of the cervical spine. Am J Surg 1939;46:494–9.
23. Brooks AL, Jenkins EB. Atlanto-axial arthrodesis by the wedge compression method. J Bone Joint Surg Am 1978;60(3):279–84.
24. Smith MD, Phillips WA, Hensinger RN. Complications of fusion to the upper cervical spine. Spine (Phila Pa 1976) 1991;16(7):702–5.

25. Coyne TJ, Fehlings MG, Wallace MC, et al. C1-C2 posterior cervical fusion: long-term evaluation of results and efficacy. Neurosurgery 1995;37(4): 688–92 [discussion: 692–3].

26. Dickman CA, Sonntag VK. Surgical management of atlantoaxial nonunions. J Neurosurg 1995;83(2): 248–53.

27. Magerl F, Seemann PS. Stable posterior fusion of the atlas and axis by transarticular screw fixation. In: Kehr P, Weidner A, editors. Cervical spine 1: Strasbourg 1985. New York: Springer-Verlag; 1987. p. 322–7.

28. Tokuhashi Y, Matsuzaki H, Shirasaki Y, et al. C1-C2 intra-articular screw fixation for atlantoaxial posterior stabilization. Spine (Phila Pa 1976) 2000;25(3):337–41.

29. Haid RW Jr, Subach BR, McLaughlin MR, et al. C1-C2 transarticular screw fixation for atlantoaxial instability: a 6-year experience. Neurosurgery 2001; 49(1):65–8 [discussion: 69–70].

30. Dickman CA, Sonntag VK. Posterior C1-C2 transarticular screw fixation for atlantoaxial arthrodesis. Neurosurgery 1998;43(2):275–80 [discussion: 280–1].

31. Song GS, Theodore N, Dickman CA, et al. Unilateral posterior atlantoaxial transarticular screw fixation. J Neurosurg 1997;87(6):851–5.

32. Grob D, Jeanneret B, Aebi M, et al. Atlanto-axial fusion with transarticular screw fixation. J Bone Joint Surg Br 1991;73(6):972–6.

33. Fuji T, Oda T, Kato Y, et al. Accuracy of atlantoaxial transarticular screw insertion. Spine (Phila Pa 1976) 2000;25(14):1760–4.

34. Apfelbaum RI. Screw fixation of the upper cervical spine: Indications and techniques. Contemp Neurosurg 1994;16(7):1–8.

35. Marcotte P, Dickman CA, Sonntag VK, et al. Posterior atlantoaxial facet screw fixation. J Neurosurg 1993;79(2):234–7.

36. Coric D, Branch CL Jr, Wilson JA, et al. Arteriovenous fistula as a complication of C1-2 transarticular screw fixation. Case report and review of the literature. J Neurosurg 1996;85(2):340–3.

37. Paramore CG, Dickman CA, Sonntag VK. The anatomical suitability of the C1-2 complex for transarticular screw fixation. J Neurosurg 1996;85(2): 221–4.

38. Harms J, Melcher RP. Posterior C1-C2 fusion with polyaxial screw and rod fixation. Spine (Phila Pa 1976) 2001;26(22):2467–71.

39. Ni B, Zhou F, Guo Q, et al. Modified technique for C1-2 screw-rod fixation and fusion using autogenous bicortical iliac crest graft. Eur Spine J 2011;8:8.

40. Stulik J, Vyskocil T, Sebesta P, et al. Atlantoaxial fixation using the polyaxial screw-rod system. Eur Spine J 2007;16(4):479–84.

41. Terterov S, Taghva A, Khalessi AA, et al. Symptomatic vertebral artery compression by the rod of a C1-C2 posterior fusion construct: case report and review of the literature. Spine (Phila Pa 1976) 2011;36(10):E678–81.

42. Plant JG, Ruff SJ. Migration of rod through skull, into brain following C1-C2 instrumental fusion for os odontoideum: a case report. Spine (Phila Pa 1976) 2010;35(3):E90–2.

43. Chun HJ, Bak KH, Kang TH, et al. Rod migration into the posterior fossa after harms operation: case report and review of literatures. J Korean Neurosurg Soc 2010;47(3):221–3.

44. Abou Madawi A, Solanki G, Casey AT, et al. Variation of the groove in the axis vertebra for the vertebral artery. Implications for instrumentation. J Bone Joint Surg Br 1997;79(5):820–3.

45. Igarashi T, Kikuchi S, Sato K, et al. Anatomic study of the axis for surgical planning of transarticular screw fixation. Clin Orthop Relat Res 2003;408(408):162–6.

46. Leonard JR, Wright NM. Pediatric atlantoaxial fixation with bilateral, crossing C-2 translaminar screws. Technical note. J Neurosurg 2006;104(Suppl 1):59–63.

Subaxial Cervical and Cervicothoracic Fixation Techniques— Indications, Techniques, and Outcomes

Miguel A. Pelton, BS[a], Joseph Schwartz, BS[b],
Kern Singh, MD[c],*

KEYWORDS

- Subaxial • Cervicothoracic • Fixation • Indications
- Techniques

The subaxial and cervicothoracic junction is a relatively difficult area for spine surgeons to navigate.[1] Because of different transitional stressors at the junction of the smaller cervical vertebrae and the larger thoracic segments, proximity to neurovascular structures, and complex anatomy, extreme care and precision must be assumed during fixation in these regions. Lateral mass screws, pedicle screws, and translaminar screws are currently the standard of choice in the subaxial cervical and upper thoracic spine.[2–5] This article addresses the relevant surgical anatomy, pitfalls, and pearls associated with each of these fixation techniques.

SURGICAL ANATOMY

The subaxial cervical spine has a lordotic posture with each vertebra composed of a body, superior and inferior articular processes, pedicles, lamina, and one spinous process. Laminae at the cervical spine are thin. Pedicles are small and are medially oriented. The facet joint is formed from superior and inferior articulating processes of the lateral masses. Orientation of the facet joint at the cervical spine is coronal in nature and prevents the spine from overextension.[1] With no articulations to the rib cage, the cervical spine allows for much more mobility than the thoracic spine.

In contrast, the upper thoracic spine has different properties due to the added elements of articulation with the thoracic rib cage. Physiologic kyphosis occurs here because of the greater height of the dorsal vertebral wall relative to the ventral vertebral surface. Moving inferiorly from C5 to T1, the height and width of the pedicles increase, with a concomitant decrease in the angle between the pedicle and vertebral body.[5] Facet joint orientation in the thoracic spine is in the coronal plane and acts to limit motion. All these elements allow for less flexion and extension than the cervical spine.

Another factor to consider in the subaxial cervical region is the uniqueness of the C7 vertebra. Often described as the transitional vertebra and representing the cervicothoracic

---

Dr Singh is a consultant for Stryker and Depuy.
[a] Department of Orthopedic Surgery, Rush University Medical Center, 1611 West Harrison Street, Chicago, IL 60612, USA
[b] Rush University Medical Center School of Medicine, 600 South Paulina Street Suite 440, Chicago, IL 60612, USA
[c] Department of Orthopedic Surgery, Rush University Medical Center, 1611 West Harrison Street, Suite 400, Chicago, IL 60612, USA
* Corresponding author.
E-mail address: kern.singh@rushortho.com

Orthop Clin N Am 43 (2012) 19–28
doi:10.1016/j.ocl.2011.08.002

junction, its small/thin lateral mass size, increased biomechanical stressors, and close proximity to neurovascular structures make the C7 vertebra a challenge during instrumentation.[6] In addition, the 5% incidence of vertebral artery passage through the transverse foramen makes avoidance of the foramen transversarium at C7 paramount during instrumentation of the pedicle and lateral mass at this level.[7]

Several muscular groups warrant knowledge of posterior fixation techniques at the cervicothoracic area. The trapezius muscle inserts medially on the spinous processes of C7 to T12. The rhomboid muscles also surround the area. The serratus posterior inferior and superior muscles are present as well as several spinal muscles that extend from the spinous processes to the transverse processes and posterior angles of the ribs. These muscles form a 6-cm to 8-cm muscular band on each side of the midline, which inserts on the underlying bony elements.[8] The neurovascular bundles rise from the intercostal vessels and the nerves run backward below the transverse process and reach the muscular layers.

Innervations of these muscles derive from the medial and lateral branches of the dorsal rami of the cervical nerves. Arterial supply to the posterior musculature inferiorly is provided by the deep cervical branch of the subclavian artery as it transverses the transverse process of C7 and the first rib. The occipital artery from the posterior external carotid supplies branches superiorly to the muscles and has branches to the vertebral and spinal arteries. The vertebral artery lies anterior to the anterior nerve roots as they exit the neural foramen. Inferiorly, the vertebral artery enters the transverse foramen at C6 and travels through each vertebral foramen through C2 where it courses posterior superior to the lateral aspect of C1. In the sagittal plane, the artery tends to move anterior in the transverse process as it runs from C6 cephalad to C2.[7]

LATERAL MASS SCREWS
Indications

Indications for lateral mass screw fixation include the following: acute and chronic instability resulting from tumors, infections, posterior element fractures, posterior ligamentous injuries, postlaminectomy instability, and following multilevel corpectomy and pseudarthrosis after anterior cervical fusion. Caution should be used in patients with abnormal bony anatomy as in those with erosive rheumatoid arthritis, osteoarthritis, or ecstatic coursing of the vertebral artery. These conditions can complicate screw placement. In cases of severe osteopenia/osteoporosis, lateral mass fixation may be supplemented with posterior wiring and/or pedicle screw fixation if the proper anatomy is present.[7]

Technique

Imaging
Fine-cut (2 mm) computed tomography (CT) with two-dimensional reconstruction and T2-weighted sagittal magnetic resonance imaging (MRI) should be used to assess lateral mass quality in the lower cervical spine.[7]

Positioning
Mayfield tongs may be used, rigidly fixing the head to the table in the prone position.[7] Gardner-Wells tongs and a face pillow can also be used.[9] Care should be taken to avoid pressure to the orbits. The neck is positioned in neutral alignment. If this might compromise spinal canal capacity to a detrimental degree, the neck is positioned flexed; an unscrubbed assistant can readjust the head holder to improve cervical lordosis after decompression once instrumentation begins. A hard collar and rotating table, such as the Jackson frame, may be used in a traumatic or severely stenotic spine to minimize cervical spine motion and increase stability during the turning process.[9] Extreme flexion or extension of the head should be avoided to prevent fusion of the neck in a nonanatomic position. Horizontal gaze may be affected if cervical alignment is not appreciated while placing instrumentation. Lateral plain radiography should be used to visualize cervical alignment.[7]

Exposures
A midline vertical skin incision can be made (as necessary) extending from the occipital protuberance past the spinous process of the seventh cervical vertebra (prominent vertebra). The nuchal ligament is divided in the midline and incised as far as the tips of the spinous processes. The deep muscle layer is stripped off the spinous processes close to the bone with the aid of electrocautery. Subperiosteral dissection is carried to the lateral boundary of the articular masses. Exposures carried too far ventrolaterally to the facet joints may result in increased bleeding and nerve root injury.[7]

Procedure
Screw insertion is located 1 mm medial to the midpoint of the lateral mass. The direction of the screw is 15° cephalad and 30° lateral for C3 to C6. Drill trajectories in the sagittal plane that are too low may violate the facet joint. Trajectories that are too medial may violate the vertebral artery.

Bicortical screw placement is recommended to ensure optimal screw anchorage. Holes are drilled with a 2.4-mm drill bit using the drill guide. Screw length should be selected 2 mm shorter than measured to avoid nerve root irritation when performing bicortical screw placement. Meticulous removal of soft tissue from the articular masses will allow for clear delineation of the anatomic landmarks. If the spinous process obstructs the application of the drill in the correct direction, it is trimmed with a rongeur. A small Penfield elevator can be placed in the joint space to keep the drill aligned in the sagittal plane parallel to the facet joint.[7]

The Roy-Camille technique may also be used for the screw entry point. The starting point for screw insertion is located at the midpoint of the lateral articular mass perpendicular to the posterior cortex of the lateral mass in the sagittal plane of the spine. The screw is directed 10° lateral with no cranial-caudal inclination (**Fig. 1**). This technique may, however, lead to cephalad articular joint violation.[7]

Magerl modified the screw placement technique by moving the starting point cephalad and medially 1 mm, then aiming 25 to 30° laterally and 45° cephalad to parallel the surface of the facet joint (**Fig. 2**).[10] An's technique uses a starting point 1 mm medial to the lateral mass center and angles the screw 30° lateral and 15° cephalad.[11] Anderson describes an alteration of the Magerl technique with a 1-mm medial offset from the center of the lateral mass with angulation of the screw 20 to 30° cephalad and 10 to 20° lateral.[9]

Auer and colleagues[9] describe the following procedure for screw and rod placement. The surgeon estimates angulation of the screw. By placing a curette or Bovie tip in the facet for visual reference, angulation of the screw can be made parallel to the facet joints. Lateral angulation can be estimated with reference to the lateral mass or by resting the drill guide on the spinous process of the next caudad level. If the spine is unstable, a high-speed 2-mm burr can be used instead of a starting awl to penetrate the lateral mass cortex. Once the outer cortex is breached, a hand drill can

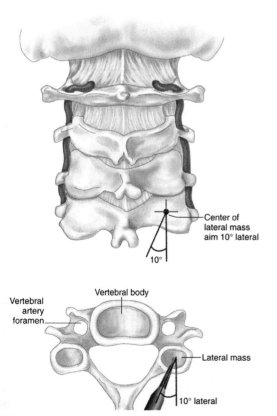

Fig. 1. Entry point and trajectory for the Roy-Camille technique. (*From* Vaccaro AR, Baron EM, Spine surgery. Operative techniques. Philadelphia: Saunders/Elsevier; 2008. p. 140; with permission.)

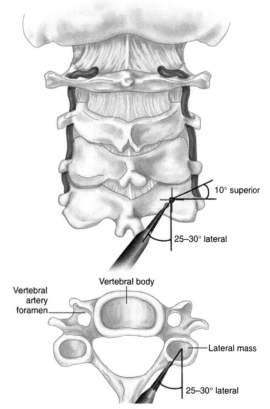

Fig. 2. Entry point and trajectory for the Magerl technique. (*From* Vaccaro AR, Baron EM, Spine surgery. Operative techniques. Philadelphia: Saunders/Elsevier; 2008. p. 141; with permission.)

be directed cephalad and lateral to the opposite side of the lateral mass. After the tapping the screw hole, the surrounding bone and the facet joint should be decorticated to maximize the fusion area. Placement at C7 can be difficult because of the angles of the posterior elements and thoracic transition. Elongation and thinning of the C7 lateral mass can also complicate screw fixation.

Minimally invasive technique

Wang and colleagues[12] describe lateral mass fixation with the following minimally invasive technique. First, a 2.0-cm midline skin incision is made to introduce a set of tubular dilator retractors after a local anesthetic. The skin entry point is chosen so that the trajectory of the tube is parallel to the facet joint in the sagittal plane approximately 2 spinal segments below the level of interest. The tube trajectory is also directed laterally to dock on the posterolateral elements and to approximate orientation using the Magerl technique. The tubular retractor diameter is 20 mm. The surface of the lateral mass is then exposed with monopolar cautery and pituitary rongeurs to remove any overlying tissues. The facet joint synovium to be fused is removed with a curette and packed with autograft bone. A cancellous drill is then used to create a 14-mm-deep pilot hole in the center of the lateral mass. The trajectory is lateral and parallel to the facet joint. The pilot hole is then tapped, and a polyaxial screw (length 14 or 16 mm, diameter 3.5 mm) is then placed under direct visualization. This is done at neighboring levels. After screw placement on one side, a connecting rod is placed down the tubular retractor and advanced into the upper polyaxial screw head using slight elevation of the tubular retractor. The procedure is then repeated on the contralateral side. Fluoroscopic guidance is used during all steps.[12]

Outcomes

Montesano[13] and Lauch demonstrated that the Magerl technique provided greater pullout resistance and a higher load to failure than the Roy-Camille technique. Choueka and colleagues[14] tested flexion failure strength and found the Magerl technique to be significantly stronger. Bicortical fixation has a potential risk of neurologic and vascular complications that range from 0.8% to 7.3%. Another study found long unicortical screws performed as well as bicortical screws. In addition, violation of the adjacent facet joint has been reported in bicortical insertion, raising the concern of extension of fusion to unintended levels. Lateral mass plating was also found to be safer with screws placed up to, but not through, the anterior lateral mass cortex while maintaining a mechanically stable construct.[7]

Nerve root injury as well as vertebral artery injury (more rare) can occur if the screw trajectory is incorrect, if penetration is too deep (bicortical screw purchase), or if there is significant past pointing of the drill. If brisk, pulsatile arterial bleeding is encountered from the drill hole, hemostasis should be obtained using bone wax, thrombogenic agents, and, potentially, placement of screw in the hole. Postoperative angiography should be obtained to determine the status of the injured vertebral artery.[7]

Auer and colleagues[9] describe lateral mass fixation as having the advantages of earlier mobilization of the patient, decreased halo brace usage, and increased fusion rates at the cervicothoracic junction. Posterior instrumentation has allowed for increased fusion rates as a result of improved bony fixation and rigidity. These techniques also have diminished immobilization time and halo bracing while maintaining the structural alignment of the spine. Lateral mass screws have expanded our ability to maintain the alignment of the spine with deficient posterior elements and multiple-level injuries.

PEDICLE SCREWS
Indications

Several studies have suggested that cervical pedicle screws are superior to the more traditional lateral mass screws when there is a need for higher pullout strength, for decreased axial load at the disk space, or for stabilization of both ventral and dorsal aspects of the spine by traversing all 3 columns of the vertebrae.[15,16] Lateral mass screws may be inadequate in cases with poor bone quality secondary to fracture, neoplasm, or revision surgery.[17] In such cases, lateral mass screws can fail by loosening or avulsion, combined with the decreasing lateral mass size at the lower cervical spine.[16]

Currently, the most accepted indications for cervical pedicle screws are: trauma-induced cervical spine fracture and dislocation; multilevel cervical instability; cervical instability after neoplasm resection; correction of cervical kyphosis; severe osteoporosis and/or absence of vertebral lamina or retrovertebral structures, making fixation difficult through other methods; and cervical instability caused by degeneration.[18]

Pedicle screws at the upper thoracic spine have many indications for a myriad of conditions. These include better pullout strength, greater control in all planes due to increased stability by 3-column fixation, fewer vertebral motion segments arthrodesed, less need for postoperative bracing, and secure fixation after laminectomy or missing posterior elements. In patients with spinal deformity, thoracic pedicle screws have been shown to have greater 3-dimensional corrections with decreased rates of curve progression and higher fusion rates.[19]

Cervical Technique

Successful placement of the screw depends on accurate entry point and trajectory. However, because the literature has not adequately established a standard approach for this, several approaches have been proposed based on healthy volunteers and cadaveric data.[20,21]

Instrumentation
Generally, screw diameters of 3.5 to 4.5 mm are used depending on pedicle size as measured by preoperative imaging. Larger diameters are needed for larger pedicles to improve fixation. For C3 to C7, the insertion point is slightly lateral to the center of the lateral mass and close to the inferior articular facet of the cephalad segment (**Figs. 3** and **4**).[7] The sagittal plane trajectory is determined by fluoroscopy or navigational guidance. The transverse plane trajectory is 25 to 45° medial. The entry site is decorticated using a burr and a high-speed drill or a rongeur. A burr or awl is used to penetrate the dorsal cortex of the pedicle.

A small curved or straight pedicle probe is used to cannulate the pedicle to develop a path for the screw through the cancellous bone of the pedicle into the vertebral body. Advancement of the probe should be smooth and consistent. A sudden plunge indicates breaking out of the pedicle laterally. An increase in resistance indicates abutment against the pedicle or vertebral body cortex.[22] After cannulation, the pedicle sounding probe is

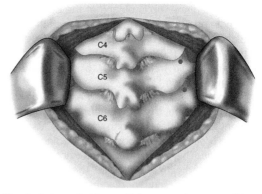

Fig. 4. Entry point for pedicle screw placement. (*From* Vaccaro AR, Baron EM, Spine surgery. Operative techniques. Philadelphia: Saunders/Elsevier; 2008. p. 153; with permission.)

placed into the pedicle, which is then palpated from within to ensure there is no medial, lateral, rostral, or caudal disruption in the cortex of the pedicles. The surgeon should listen carefully to the sound of the cannulation to make sure that the integrity of the ventral cortex is intact and it is not being penetrated by the pilot hole.

Minimally invasive technique
The desired surgical level is identified via lateral fluoroscopy or plain radiography. The starting point is 2 to 3 cm lateral to the midline. Adjunctive anteroposterior views allow for precise determination for the starting position in the transverse plane. A guidewire is inserted under fluoroscopy in 2 perpendicular planes up to the rostral lamina of the facet joint at the desired level. Next, a 2-cm incision is made around the Kirschner wire and sequential dilators are used down to the posterior spinal elements.[23]

Upper Thoracic Technique

Meticulous exposure of the posterior elements is required.[19] The inferior 3 to 5 mm of the inferior facet is osteotomized and articular cartilage on the dorsal side of the superior facet is completely removed except for the lowest instrumented vertebra. Typically, the starting point is more lateral and caudad at the T1 to T2 level than the lower thoracic spine. A burr is used to create a posterior cortical breach. The pedicle blush may be visualized suggesting entrance into the cancellous bone of the pedicle. With appropriate ventral pressure, the thoracic gearshift is placed into the base of the pedicle and initially pointed laterally to avoid medial wall perforation. After insertion of the gearshift by approximately 15 to 20 mm, the gearshift is removed and the tip is turned to face medially.

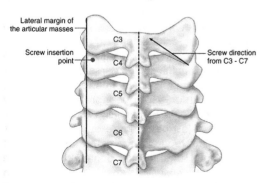

Fig. 3. Entry point for pedicle screw placement. (*From* Vaccaro AR, Baron EM, Spine surgery. Operative techniques. Philadelphia: Saunders/Elsevier; 2008. p. 153; with permission.)

The pedicle finder tip is placed at the base of the prior hole and then inserted down the path of the pedicle medially to a depth of 30 to 35 mm. Rotation of the finder by 180° makes room for the screw. A transverse angle trajectory of 15° is acceptable for screw insertion.[19]

The pedicle seeker is removed and the tract is visualized to see that no cerebrospinal fluid is present. A flexible palpating device is used to palpate 5 distinct bony borders, including a floor and 4 walls. Then the length of the tract is marked and measured with a hemostat. The pedicle tract is undertapped using a diameter 1.0 mm less than that of the intended screw (eg, 4.5-mm tap for a 5.5-mm screw). The screw is inserted into the pedicle, into the body in the same alignment to confirm it is threaded properly and allow for viscoelastic expansion. Confirmation occurs via intraoperative anterioposterior and lateral fluoroscopy.[19]

Outcomes and Evidence

Pedicle screw fixation has also demonstrated positive clinical outcomes in the reconstruction of metastatic lesions of the spine.[17] In this retrospective review of 32 patients who underwent palliative spinal reconstruction for metastatic spinal tumors with cervical pedicle screws, all had an improvement of neck pain. In addition, 24 (83%) of the 29 patients with spinal cord lesions demonstrated neurologic improvement, and 16 of 18 nonambulatory patients became ambulatory after screw fixation. Of great significance in the study was that posterior decompression followed by pedicle screw fixation provided significant neural decompression in 78% of patients.[17] Thus, fixation at the subaxial level seems a valid and reliable method for metastatic tumors.

The usage of pedicle screws is not always straightforward, however, especially when it comes to the complex biomechanical forces at C7 vertebra.[6] One cadaveric study assessed the use of either pedicle screws or lateral mass screws at C7 with treatment of lateral mass screws at C4 to C6 beforehand in 10 cadaveric specimens. After measuring the motion of C4 with respect to C7 in flexion and extension and lateral bending in a materials testing machine, lateral mass screws and pedicle screws showed no significant differences in postcyclical flexion-extension and lateral bending.[6] As suggested by this study, with the complex biomechanical loads and higher chances for damage to neurovascular structures at C7, lateral mass screws, at least in vitro, might be the better choice.[6] Further clinical studies at the C7 vertebra are needed to verify this claim.

TRANSLAMINAR SCREWS
Indications

Although pedicle screw usage in the subaxial cervical spine is widely accepted, because of the relatively short height of the pedicle at T1, and the proximity of T1 and T2 to the superior and inferior nerve roots, its application is more challenging in the upper thoracic spine. The lack of epidural space and increased medial angulation needed for pedicle cannulation also increase the chances of damage to adjacent neural structures.[24,25] In 2006, Kretzer and colleagues[25] reported the first use of translaminar screws in the upper thoracic spine and mentioned that the advantages over pedicle screw placement justify its usage in certain cases. Easier visualization of high thoracic lamina following standard posterior exposure allows the dorsal side of the lamina to serve as a guide for the subsequent screw placement trajectory. This is in contrast with pedicle screw placement where the surgeon needs to place the screw without direct visualization of the pedicle.

The most current indications for translaminar screws in the upper thoracic spine based on limited literature and experience are degenerative disease, neoplasm, trauma, and, most recently, for stabilization of the pediatric upper thoracic spine.[24–26] In addition, translaminar screw usage at the cervical spine has been well established particularly at the C2 level.

Technique

Instrumentation
Screw width ranges from 3.5 to 4.5 mm. Screw length is at least 25 mm at T1 and at least 20 mm at T2.[24]

Procedure
Entry is at the contralateral spinolaminar junction (base of the spinous process) and the target is the junction of the transverse process and the superior facet contralateral to the entry point. The trajectory is approximately the slope of the contralateral lamina angled dorsally to avoid violation of the ventral laminar cortex. The hole is palpated with a ball-tipped probe, and screw placement follows sequentially. The same procedure occurs for the opposite spinolaminar junction. Titanium rods are contoured and cut to the appropriate length and tightened with the concomitant cervical segment. Fusion with an autograft or allograft can follow from cervical segment to T1/T2. Intraoperative plain radiography verifies correct positioning of the construct (**Figs. 5** and **6**).[24]

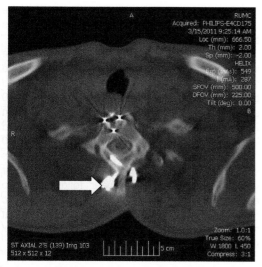

Fig. 5. Axial CT scan of translaminar screw fixation at T1 (*arrow*).

Outcomes

As noted previously, the literature on the use of translaminar screws at the upper thoracic spine is scant.[24–26] Kretzer and colleagues[24] analyzed the use of translaminar screws for inferior fixation across the cervicothoracic junction and found them to be only useful in cases where the posterior elements of spinous processes and lamina are intact. This includes patients with smaller pedicles on preoperative CT scans. The study showed that this technique of fixation is not without risks and flaws. Because the ventral laminar wall is not readily visualized in screw placement, penetration

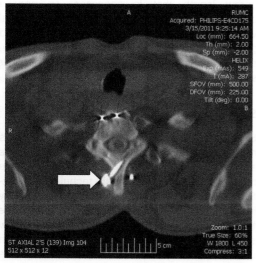

Fig. 6. Axial CT scan of translaminar screw fixation at T1 (*arrow*).

must be avoided here as damage could occur to the thecal sac or spinal cord. In addition, translaminar screw placement depends on an intact pedicle for transmission of forces throughout the vertebral body.[24] To date, no long-term studies have evaluated the complications, if any, of the translaminar approach.

In a follow-up study, Kretzer and colleagues[25] used CT to retrospectively assess 100 patients (50 men and 50 women) for differences in diameter, maximal screw length, and optimal screw trajectory for translaminar screw placement at T1 to T2 and compared the results with the same parameters for pedicle screws. They reported that pedicle screws also differed between the T1 and T2 vertebrae. In addition, male patients were able to tolerate longer translaminar screws at T1 and at T2 compared with female patients.[25] Thus, future clinical outcomes may also depend on sex.[25] With the improved insertional torque/pullout strengths relative to pedicle screws at the same position, translaminar screws seem to be the better choice for stability at the upper thoracic spine.[25]

In addition, translaminar fixation seems to be a valid technique for pediatric cases over pedicle screws. Recently, Patel and colleagues[26] analyzed the outcomes of translaminar screws in the pediatric population. The study analyzed 130 consecutive CT scans of the upper thoracic spines of 70 boys and 60 girls and analyzed them by laminar height and thickness, screw length, and screw angle. In accordance with Ketzer and colleagues,[26] the researchers found that there were significant differences in mean laminar height, screw length, and screw angle at isolated angles when comparing the male and female patients. Moreover, the investigators found that the anatomy of the upper thoracic spine does not limit the use of translaminar screws in most pediatric patients. Thus, translaminar screw placement seems a suitable alternative to avoid the dangers associated with pedicle screw placement in children, namely, because of the small size of the pedicles, proximity to critical structures, and the increased risk for neurovascular damage.

COMPLICATIONS
Lateral Mass Screws

One recent study specifically analyzed the complications of 1662 lateral mass screw fixations in 3 subcategories: intraoperative, early (within a week), and late complications (within 1 year).[27] Intraoperative complications included fracture of the lateral mass in 27 (1.6%) screws, and bicortical screw-associated radiculopathy in 3 patients

(1.3%). Early complications comprised 2 cases (0.8%) of postoperative hematoma and 5 cases (2.2%) of deltoid muscle weakness.[27] All these early complications resolved within 5 months of the initial operation without surgical correction of screw placement.[27] Late complications included screw pullout in 3 patients (1.3%), pseudarthrosis in 6 cases (2.6%), and reoperations in 14 cases (6.2%).[27] Significantly, no cases of vertebral artery injury, dural tears, superficial or deep infections, hardware breakage, or death were noted.[27] These low complication rates and improved clinical outcomes suggest that lateral mass screws at the subaxial spine are a safe and viable fixation technique.

Screw placement may be difficult in patients with aberrant bony anatomy, such as those with rheumatoid arthritis or advanced osteoarthritis, or in patients with an ecstatic coursing of the vertebral artery.[7] In the former case, arthritic changes may result in inadequate screw purchase for sufficient stabilization. In such cases, supplementation with posterior wiring and/or pedicle screw fixation may be indicated.[7] These cases may also require rigid external fixation with a postoperative halo-vest orthosis.[7]

Complications may also occur if inappropriate screw trajectories and insertions are chosen. Screw trajectories that are too far medial and too deep can injure the vertebral artery and warrant the need for hemostasis with bone wax and thrombogenic agents.[7] Screw insertion drill trajectories in the sagittal plane that are too low may violate the facet joint. This can be avoided by placing a Penfield elevator in the joint space to keep the drill aligned in the sagittal plane parallel to the facet joint.[7]

Wang and colleagues[12] reported on 18 consecutive patients with the minimally invasive technique and found that postoperative CT scans showed no cases of screw misplacement and fusion occurred successfully in all patients without changes in sagittal alignment. The only complication reported in the study was a change to the open technique in 2 patients because of large body habitus that prevented caudal screw insertion.[12]

Pedicle Screws

Cervical pedicle screw fixation at the subaxial cervical and upper thoracic spine also has a significant risk of neurovascular complications. These can occur especially in patients with insufficient pedicles (<4.5 mm in diameter, destruction of pedicles by trauma/tumor), and in those with a single dominant vertebral artery.[7] In these cases,

the pedicle cannot support a screw and the danger of injury to the vertebral artery increases significantly.

Kim and colleagues[28] specifically assessed the safety and potential complications of pedicle screws at the upper thoracic spine. They found that out of 577 pedicle screw insertions, 10 showed medial cortical wall violation between 2.5 and 5.0 mm and 26 screw insertions showed lateral cortical perforation between 3.0 and 6.0 mm. However, none of these screw violations showed any subsequent signs of neurologic or vascular symptoms at 10-year follow-up.[28] To avoid the chance of any possible neurologic complications, the investigators hypothesize that a "definite safe zone" of less than 2 mm medial encroachment should be respected.[28]

Translaminar Screws

Complications of translaminar screw fixations at the upper thoracic spine and C2 vertebrae have not been extensively studied. Dorward and Wright[29] most recently reported on a series of 103 C2 translaminar screw placements and found no cases of vascular or neurologic injuries and only 1 case of pseudoarthrosis/instrumentation failure. Kretzer and colleagues[25] reported on upper thoracic translaminar screw fixation and stated that complications can occur because the ventral laminar wall cannot be visualized, and can thus be penetrated and lead to damage to the thecal sac or the spinal cord. This can be avoided by dorsal angulation as judged by the slope of the dorsal laminar surface during intralaminar drilling.[25] Neurologic damage can also be avoided by preoperative axial CT scans to estimate the screw length that is necessary to provide adequate bone purchase and to avoid cortical violation.[25] More studies in both the adult and pediatric populations will elucidate more, if any, complications that can occur in translaminar screw fixation.

SUMMARY

Subaxial and cervicothoracic fixation techniques represent a unique challenge to practicing spine surgeons. Lateral mass screws still represent the most cohesive and appropriate technique for fixation at the subaxial spine from C3 to C7, especially in cases with missing posterior elements. At the transitional level of C7, the lateral mass screw seems to be the most appropriate for fixation unless the vertebral artery courses through the C7 transverse foramen and if C7 is not large enough for pedicle insertion.

Pedicle mass screws are indicated at the subaxial spine when there is a need for better pullout strength. Translaminar screws are acceptable for fixation at the upper cervical and upper thoracic (C2, T1, and T2) spine in both adults and children because of the superior visualization of the lamina and the lesser risk of neurovascular compromise involved in their usage. Minimally invasive surgical techniques with these screw types are on the increase to reduce postoperative pain and improve clinical outcomes. With more surgeons practicing the techniques outlined in this article and more studies analyzing the minimally invasive techniques, subaxial and cervicothoracic spine fixation procedures will be further refined and improved.

REFERENCES

1. Lapsiwala S, Benzel E. Surgical management of cervical myelopathy dealing with the cervical-thoracic junction. Spine J 2006;6(Suppl 6):268S–73S.
2. An HS, Coppes MA. Posterior cervical fixation for fracture and degenerative disc disease. Clin Orthop Relat Res 1997;(335):101–11.
3. Anderson PA, Henley MB, Grady MS, et al. Posterior cervical arthrodesis with AO reconstruction plates and bone graft. Spine (Phila Pa 1976) 1991; 16(Suppl 3):S72–9.
4. Heller JG, Carlson GD, Abitbol JJ, et al. Anatomic comparison of the Roy-Camille and Magerl techniques for screw placement in the lower cervical spine. Spine (Phila Pa 1976) 1991;16(Suppl 10):S552–7.
5. Wang VY, Chou D. The cervicothoracic junction. Neurosurg Clin N Am 2007;18(2):365–71.
6. Xu R, McGirt MJ, Sutter EG, et al. Biomechanical comparison between C-7 lateral mass and pedicle screws in subaxial cervical constructs. Presented at the 2009 Joint Spine Meeting. Laboratory investigation. J Neurosurg Spine 2010;13(6):688–94.
7. Vaccaro AR, Baron EM. Spine surgery. Operative techniques. Philadelphia: Saunders/Elsevier; 2008. xviii. p. 481.
8. Aebi M, Arlet V, Webb JK. APspine manual. Dubendorf (NY): AOSpine International; Thieme (distributor); 2007. p. 837.
9. Auer BP, Alander DH. Posterior instrumentation of the subaxial cervical spine. Contemporary Spine Surgery 2006;7(8):1–6.
10. Jeanneret B, Gebhard JS, Magerl F. Transpedicular screw fixation of articular mass fracture-separation: results of an anatomical study and operative technique. J Spinal Disord 1994;7(3):222–9.
11. An HS, Gordin R, Renner K. Anatomic considerations for plate-screw fixation of the cervical spine. Spine 1991;16:S548–51.
12. Wang MY, Levi AD. Minimally invasive lateral mass screw fixation in the cervical spine: initial clinical experience with long-term follow-up. Neurosurgery 2006;58(5):907–12 [discussion: 907–12].
13. Montesano PX, Jauch E, Jonsson H Jr. Anatomic and biomechanical study of posterior cervical plate arthrodesis: an evaluation of two different techniques of screw placement. J Spinal Disord 1992;5:301–5.
14. Muffoletto AJ, Yang J, Vadhva M, et al. Cervical stability with lateral mass plating: unicortical versus bicortical screw purchase. Spine (Phila Pa 1976) 2003;28(8):778–81.
15. Johnston TL, Karaikovic EE, Lautenschlager EP, et al. Cervical pedicle screws vs. lateral mass screws: uniplanar fatigue analysis and residual pullout strengths. Spine J 2006;6(6):667–72.
16. Hong JT, Tomoyuki T, Udayakumar R, et al. Biomechanical comparison of three different types of C7 fixation techniques. Spine (Phila Pa 1976) 2011; 36(5):393–8.
17. Oda I, Abumi K, Ito M, et al. Palliative spinal reconstruction using cervical pedicle screws for metastatic lesions of the spine: a retrospective analysis of 32 cases. Spine (Phila Pa 1976) 2006;31(13):1439–44.
18. Liu Y, Hu JH, Yu KY. Pedicle screw fixation for cervical spine instability: clinical efficacy and safety analysis. Chin Med J (Engl) 2009;122(17):1985–9.
19. Kim YJ, Lenke LG. Thoracic pedicle screw placement: free-hand technique. Neurol India 2005;53(4):512–9.
20. Zheng X, Chaudhari R, Wu C, et al. Subaxial cervical pedicle screw insertion with newly defined entry point and trajectory: accuracy evaluation in cadavers. Eur Spine J 2010;19(1):105–12.
21. Rao RD, Marawar SV, Stemper BD, et al. Computerized tomographic morphometric analysis of subaxial cervical spine pedicles in young asymptomatic volunteers. J Bone Joint Surg Am 2008;90(9): 1914–21.
22. Benzel EC. Spine surgery: techniques, complication avoidance, and management. 2nd edition. Philadelphia: Churchill Livingstone; 2005.
23. Denaro L, D'Avella D, Denaro V, et al. Pitfalls in cervical spine surgery avoidance and management of complications. Berlin and Heidelberg: Springer-Verlag; 2010.
24. Kretzer RM, Chaput C, Sciubba DM, et al. A computed tomography-based feasibility study of translaminar screw fixation in the upper thoracic spine. J Neurosurg Spine 2010;12(3):286–92.
25. Kretzer RM, Sciubba DM, Bagley CA, et al. Translaminar screw fixation in the upper thoracic spine. J Neurosurg Spine 2006;5(6):527–33.
26. Patel AJ, Cherian J, Fulkerson DH, et al. Computed tomography morphometric analysis for translaminar screw fixation in the upper thoracic spine of the pediatric population. J Neurosurg Pediatr 2011; 7(4):383–8.

27. Katonis P, Papadakis SA, Galanakos S, et al. Lateral mass screw complications: analysis of 1662 screws. J Spinal Disord Tech 2010. [Epub ahead of print].

28. Kim YJ, Lenke LG, Bridwell KH, et al. Free hand pedicle screw placement in the thoracic spine: is it safe? Spine (Phila Pa 1976) 2004;29(3):333–42 [discussion: 342].

29. Dorward IG, Wright NM. Seven years of experience with c2 translaminar screw fixation: clinical series and review of the literature. Neurosurgery 2011; 68(6):1491–9.

Posterior Surgery for Cervical Myelopathy: Indications, Techniques, and Outcomes

Brandon D. Lawrence, MD*, Darrel S. Brodke, MD

KEYWORDS

- Cervical • Spondylotic • Myelopathy • Laminectomy
- Laminoplasty • Fusion

Cervical spondylosis is the most common cause of acquired disability in patients over the age of 50 and cervical spondylotic myelopathy (CSM) is the most common progressive spinal cord disorder in patients over the age of 55.[1] Despite this, controversy remains in the literature regarding the optimal treatment regimen and optimal timing of treatment when caring for patients with CSM, particularly when the disease process is in its early stages.[1] This is likely due to the paucity of well-designed prospective studies with validated outcome measures that clearly delineate patient populations and identify the best course of treatment.

Surgical treatments to decompress the neural elements in patients with CSM that is moderate to severe (modified Japanese Orthopaedic Association [mJOA] score <12) or progressive in nature have been shown to significantly improve functional status and pain when compared with non-operatively treated patients.[2] Nonoperative modalities, however, have shown maintenance of or even improvement in functional status in patients under 75 years old with mild CSM (mJOA score >12).[3] Nonoperative treatment modalities should be entertained before embarking on surgical decompression in patients with mild CSM. Even though the traditional natural history of myelopathic patients is a slow, stepwise decline, there is a subset of patients who maintain a steady state without

further neurologic decline with nonoperative treatment.[4] Conversely, there is a subset of patients who have shown benefit from surgical decompression even in the setting of mild myelopathy, and factors associated with stabilization/improvement of functional outcomes include advanced age, long duration of symptoms, and/or rapid progression of symptoms.[5]

Additionally, controversy exists surrounding the optimal surgical approach for patients with CSM: anterior versus posterior decompression. Both have been shown beneficial. Typically, the anterior approach is used when shorter decompressions are required and the posterior approach is used when longer (3+ segment) decompressions are needed. Regardless of the approach, the goal of surgery in myelopathic patients is adequate decompression of the neural elements to halt progression of symptoms and improve patient symptomology. This article discusses in detail the techniques, outcomes, and associated complications for each of 3 specific techniques used to treat cervical myelopathy from a posterior approach.

INCIDENCE AND ETIOLOGY

The true incidence of CSM at present is unknown yet it remains the most common cause of spinal cord dysfunction in patients over the age of 55.[1] This is likely due to the subtle findings in patients

The authors have nothing to disclose.
Department of Orthopaedics, University of Utah, 590 Wakara Way, Salt Lake City, UT 84108, USA
* Corresponding author.
E-mail address: brandon.lawrence@hsc.utah.edu

Orthop Clin N Am 43 (2012) 29–40
doi:10.1016/j.ocl.2011.09.003

living with mild myelopathy or patients not seeking care. What is known is that as the population ages and life spans increase the incidence of patients presenting with CSM will likely continue to rise.

CSM is a clinical diagnosis made by identifying long-tract signs in the upper and lower extremities and is largely a result of direct mechanical compression on the spinal cord. Compressive effects on the spinal cord have a multitude of causes, grouped as static or dynamic factors. Static factors represent narrowing of the spinal canal secondary to acquired conditions (eg, spondylosis) and/or developmental conditions (eg, congenitally narrow canal).[6] Dynamic factors, such as segmental vertebral instability, also play a role in spinal cord compression and may aggravate the underlying static factors, resulting in repetitive cord compression and neurologic injury.[7] Additionally, Breig and colleagues[8] have shown that morphologic changes occur within the spinal cord with flexion and extension that may also play a role in the development of myelopathy. As the cervical spine flexes the spinal cord stretches and it may be prone to pathologic compression if it abuts spondylotic changes ventrally. As the cervical spine extends the spinal cord thickens and it may be prone to pathologic compression as the ligamentum flavum infolds or it may abut the lamina in congenitally stenotic patients.

The static and dynamic factors that cause spinal cord compression may have additive affects that cause reversible (mild–moderate myelopathy) and irreversible (severe myelopthy) damage to the neurons, axons, and glial cells of the spinal cord. Histologic studies on autopsy specimens have shown loss of neurons and vacuolar degeneration in the gray matter along with demyelination, myelin fragmentation, and swelling of the axons in white matter.[9,10]

PHYSICAL EXAMINATION AND IMAGING

Patients presenting with myelopathy often complain of issues with balance, gait disturbances, and loss of fine motor skill and hand dexterity. These symptoms are often first noted by family members who notice a wide-based gait and a diminishing ability to use buttons or zippers. Patients may also complain of urinary urgency, frequency, and/or hesitation but rarely note incontinence. Axially based neck pain and radicular symptoms are also common concomitant complaints.

Signs of myelopathy on physical examination include gait instability, positive Romberg sign, hyperreflexia, inverted radial reflex, Hoffmann signs, pathologic clonus, and upgoing toes on plantar stimulation. Ono and colleagues[11] described a characteristic dysfunction of the hand that was observed in patients with cervical spinal cord compression. They noted loss of power of adduction, extension of the ulnar 2 or 3 fingers, and an inability to grip and release rapidly with these fingers. Ono and colleagues[11] termed these changes, *myelopathy hand*, which seemed due to pyramidal tract involvement. Changes in pain, temperature, and proprioception may also be noted. If spinal cord compression is present above the C3 level, a scapulohumeral reflex may be noted.

Depending on the level of suspicion and magnitude of presenting signs/symptoms, advanced imaging may be necessary. In the absence of any red flags (tumor, trauma, infection, and/or neurologic injury), the acquisition of upright plain radiographs, including dynamic flexion/extension views, is recommended initially. If red flags are present, advanced imaging (CT and/or MRI) should proceed without delay.

Plain radiography may portray evidence of spondylotic changes, including disk space collapse, uncovertebral joint hypertrophy, facet arthropathy, and vertebral endplate sclerosis but the commonality of these findings should be kept in mind. The presence of an ossified posterior longitudinal ligament (OPLL), congenital stenosis, or dynamic instability may be more diagnostic in relation to myelopathy.

MRI remains the gold standard in evaluating the soft tissues of the cervical spine, including the disks, ligaments, and neural elements. Because of the sensitivity of MRI in visualizing abnormalities of the soft tissues, it is important to correlate MRI findings with patients' signs/symptoms.[12] Intramedullary spinal cord changes on MRI have been correlated with histopathological findings by Ohshio and colleagues.[13] They described abnormally high T2-weighted image signal intensities that appeared nonspecifically in mildly altered lesions or areas with edema. These lesions may resolve with time. A more ominous finding is when a low T1-weighted image in addition to a high T2-weighted image signal intensity appears in the gray matter. This represents severely altered lesions with necrosis, myelomalacia, or spongiform change. Additionally, abnormally high T1-weighted image intensities in the white matter also appear in severely altered lesions.

Currently, the findings of cord signal changes on MRI cannot be correlated with either the prognosis of patients with CSM or their outcome if operative decompression is elected.[14,15] There are ongoing studies looking at diffusion tensor MRI sequences in hopes of not only providing prognostic and outcome data but also delineating the timing of intervention controversy that exists today.[16]

When evaluating patients with CSM, CT scanning with myelography plays a vital role, especially if contraindications to performing an MRI scan exist (pacemaker, foreign bodies, and so forth). Even though CT myelograms are an invasive procedure, they delineate osseous sources of compression from soft tissue sources that may not be well visualized on MRI scanning, as seen in the setting of OPLL. Shafaie and colleagues[17] compared the inter-rater reliability between CT myelography and MRI scanning and found it only moderately good. The investigators tended to more severely grade the degree of central and neuroforaminal stenosis with CT myelogram, which more clearly delineated the osseous pathology. They concluded that CT myelogram and MRI are complementary studies not exclusive studies.

RATIONALE AND OPTIONS FOR POSTERIOR DECOMPRESSION

When considering surgical options in the treatment of patients with CSM, the principle goal is adequate decompression of the neural elements. The key factors to consider when deciding which approach is best suited for a patient are the number of levels requiring decompression, the cervical sagittal alignment, whether or not the anterior cervical spine is ankylosed (ankylosing spondylitis or diffuse idiopathic skeletal hyperostosis), the presence of OPLL, the presence of dynamic instability, and the anatomic location of the compressive structures.

The anterior approach is most commonly used when there are 3 or fewer levels involved, cervical lordosis has been lost, the spine is not ankylosed, or if dynamic instability is present. In patients with OPLL and severe compression (>60% canal compromise), it has been shown that anterior decompression via corpectomy has improved neurologic recovery but has increased complications associated with the anterior approach[18] and may have increased risk of dural injury. The posterior approach should be considered.

The posterior approach is best suited when 3 or more levels are involved, when cervical lordosis is preserved, when the spine is ankylosed, and possibly in the setting of OPLL (discussed previously).[19,20] Cervical sagittal alignment is crucial to note because a posterior decompression in a kyphotic cervical spine does not allow the spinal cord to migrate posteriorly and, if the kyphosis progresses, further compression on the cord may ensue causing worsening neurologic decline.[21] Within this subset, there are 3 possible techniques discussed in detail: (1) decompressive laminectomy alone, (2) laminectomy and fusion, and (3) laminoplasty.

POSTERIOR TECHNIQUES FOR CERVICAL MYELOPATHY
Decompressive Laminectomy

Historically, laminectomy has been successfully used to treat CSM, with many case series showing successful outcomes. Posterior decompression was and is largely reserved for multilevel stenosis, with one- and two-level disease treated anteriorly. The standard laminectomy length is 3 to 5 levels, because this allows room for the spinal cord to migrate away from anterior structures in addition to removing dorsal compression. The concern with removal of this number of laminae and spinous processes without concomitant fusion is the loss of stability, allowing late kyphotic collapse.

The literature on laminectomy for CSM is replete with level-3 evidence and little evidence above this level. There has emerged a clear expectation for modest improvement in some patients treated in this fashion with loss of that improvement in a subset of patients. Arnold and colleagues[22] found an initial 77% improvement in neurologic status, although at late (8-year) follow-up, that was maintained in only 52% of patients. Likewise, Bishara[23] reported improvement in 56% of the 59 patients in their report at 5 years, which dropped to 51% improvement at the 10-year follow-up, with no reported instability in any of the patients. Carol and Ducker[24] reported somewhat better long-term improvement rates. They evaluated 125 patients who underwent laminectomy compared with another 81 patients who underwent anterior decompression and fusion and 10 patients with combined approaches. The laminectomy group compared favorably with 68% improvement rate at a mean 10-year follow-up. Kato and colleagues,[25] like the other investigators, reported an early recovery rate better than long-term improvement. They found a 44% recovery rate 1 year after laminectomy, although by 10 years, this had been maintained in only 32.8% of the 44 patients followed.

Over the past several decades, this technique has fallen out of favor, largely because of the increased rate of complications in comparison with other surgical techniques. Postlaminectomy kyphosis is the most concerning complication and seems to occur in 10% to 45% of patients. Matsunaga and colleagues[26] compared 37 patients treated by laminectomy alone with 64 patients who underwent laminoplasty, with a mean follow-up of greater than 5 years. They found postoperative kyphosis rates of 35% in the laminectomy group and only 7% in the laminoplasty group. Likewise, Kato and colleagues[25] found 47% of patients developed postoperative kyphosis, although this did not correlate with neurologic deterioration. Perez-Lopez and colleagues[27] found a 24% rate of postlaminectomy kyphosis in the 19 patients who underwent laminectomy compared with only 7% in the 17 who underwent laminectomy and fusion, whereas Hamanishi and Tanaka[28] found a postoperative kyphosis rate of only 17% of the 35 patients who underwent laminectomy alone and no difference from the fusion group.[28] They did select those deemed to have preoperative instability to fusion, so the 2 groups were not comparable.

The rate of postlaminectomy kyphosis seems to increase in patients with straightened or kyphotic spines preoperatively. The risk may be lower in patients with advanced degenerative changes, fully collapsed disks, and decreased motion in the cervical spine. Postlaminectomy kyphosis may lead to further neurologic deterioration.

Patients with multiroot radiculopathy tend to do less well with laminectomy alone.[29] This may in part be because of the hesitation to remove too much facet if a fusion is not planned, for fear of creating instability. A more significant facetectomy is often required to adequately decompress the roots, so decompressive laminectomy alone is not the correct procedure when significant foraminal decompression is needed.

Other common complications of decompressive laminectomy for CSM include immediate neurologic loss, progressive long-term neurologic deterioration, hematoma, and wound infection. In an extensive review of 310 patients having undergone laminectomy over a 6-year time period, Halvorsen and colleagues[30] report that 11.6% of patients deteriorated in their neurologic function immediately after surgery, 41.2% improved in function, and 47.2% were unchanged in neurologic function. More than half of the patients who experienced neurologic loss postoperatively had permanent changes. At final follow-up, only half of the patients undergoing laminectomy for CSM had improvement in their neurologic status. This is similar to other studies (discussed previously), with better early results and progressive loss of that improvement at 5-year to 10-year follow-up.[22,23,25] Rates of postoperative hematoma are approximately 1% and are more likely in those patients with prior surgery,[30] and postoperative wound infections occur in approximately 1% to 4% of patients after laminectomy.[30,31]

In response to this concern of postlaminectomy kyphosis and progressive long-term loss of neurologic improvement, Yukawa and colleagues[32] reported on a skip laminectomy technique and prospectively randomized 41 CSM patients to this technique or laminoplasty. Although only short-term (1-year) results are reported to date, they show no differences between groups. This technique may work well if the spine is neutral to lordotic, most of the compression is dorsal, and some dorsal migration of the cord is not required.

Multilevel laminectomy has been a long-used technique for decompressing the spinal cord in patients with CSM. Modest success rates are similar to other techniques, although with a moderate rate of late loss of neurologic improvement and postlaminectomy kyphosis, this technique has become less popular than the others covered in this review.

Laminectomy with Fusion

Given the rate of late neurologic deterioration and the moderate rate of postlaminectomy kyphosis (discussed previously), the concept of performing a posterior cervical fusion at the time of decompression gained interest. Early techniques included onlay bone grafting after decompressive laminectomy. Because of the increased risks of pseudoarthrosis and early kyphotic collapse after onlay bone grafting techniques in the posterior cervical spine, most surgeons advocate for a posterior instrumented fusion because it provides secure stabilization, does not interfere with decompression, and permits early mobilization of the patient.[33] There are several techniques used for instrumented posterior cervical fusion, including sublaminar/facet wiring techniques as well as pedicle/lateral mass screw-rod techniques, but the latter is yet to be approved by the Food and Drug Administration. Pedicle/lateral mass screw-rod placement, however, is favorable due to ease of placement as well as providing rigid segmental fixation in the setting of a wide posterior laminectomy/foraminotomy. This is now the most common technique used for posterior stabilization.

The operative technique for the placement of screws in the posterior cervical spine typically involves the placement of pedicle screws/pars screws at C2, lateral mass screws at C3 through C6, and pedicle screws at C7 and below. Given the complex and variable neurovascular anatomy of the cervical spine, it is recommended that all patients undergo imaging studies to assess the neurovascular anatomy before applying posterior cervical screws for fixation.

Placement of lateral mass screws was initially described by Roy-Camille and Saillant[34] with a recommendation to place the screws in a direction perpendicular to the lamina starting at the midpoint of the lamina. This technique was later modified by Magerl[35] in an effort to increase length of fixation and improve the safety and efficacy of screw placement to avoid the exiting nerve root (by aiming cephalad) and the vertebral artery (by aiming laterally). Their recommendations were to start slightly superiorly and medially to the midpoint of the lamina and aim 25° degrees and 45° in the cephalad direction. Several anatomic studies have been performed with reports of the Magerl[35] technique having a higher incidence of potential nerve root injury[36] and another study stating that the Roy-Camille technique is safer at C3 and C4 and the Magerl technique at C5 and C6 because of the varying angles of the facet joints.[37] Both techniques were described with bicortical fixation and, with the use of locked polyaxial screws commonly used today, most surgeons place these unicortically to minimize the risk of nerve root injury while maintaining fixation strength (**Fig. 1**).

Many small cases series with short follow-up of CSM patients treated by cervical laminectomy and fusion have been published. They all reveal a neurologic improvement rate of 75% to 90%, better than generally seen in the laminectomy literature. Those studies directly comparing decompressive laminectomy with concomitant posterior instrumented fusion to laminectomy have shown superiority of fusion to laminectomy alone in regards to preventing late neurologic deterioration and postlaminectomy kyphosis (described previously). But, laminectomy with instrumented fusion is not without its own inherent complications. Pseudoarthrosis rates have dropped from more than 35%[38] in the early literature[39] to 2.7% with modern instrumentation techniques in patients with CSM.[40] Fusion of the cervical spine alters the biomechanical environment and when axial and rotational loads are altered over several segments the force distribution through the cervical spine may be shifted to the adjacent levels, resulting in adjacent segment degeneration.[38,41]

Additional complications include those specifically related to hardware placement. Graham and colleagues[42] discussed complications of lateral mass screw placement using the Magerl technique and reported a 6.1% incidence of malpositioned screws in 21 patients. Three patients developed radicular symptoms that warranted revision of the hardware and therefore had a 1.8% per-screw risk of radiculopathy. There were no vertebral artery or spinal cord injuries; all patients had evidence of radiographic union; and there were no implant failures. More recently, Katonis and colleagues[40] analyzed 225 patients and 1662 lateral mass screws and reported intraoperative

fracture of the lateral mass in 27 screws as well as nerve root irritation in 3 bicortically placed screws that required repositioning. They reported no vertebral artery or spinal cord injuries and a 2.7% pseudarthrosis rate with screw pullout in 3 cases with a mean follow-up of 18 months.

Laminectomy and fusion seems to combine the early improvement in neurologic function seen with decompressive laminectomy with less late loss of function or kyphotic collapse and with a lower overall complication rate. It has become the standard surgical treatment of patients with CSM due to multilevel stenosis and cord compression, to which other treatments are most commonly compared.[43–45]

Laminoplasty

Because of the complications of decompressive laminectomy alone and several reports of poor outcomes with laminectomy and fusion in the Japanese population, the concept of laminoplasty evolved.[43,46,47] With this concept of expansive cervical laminoplasties, many different techniques in performing a laminoplasty have been described. Advocates for this technique think that this procedure preserves stability while maintaining motion, therefore decreasing the risk of adjacent segment degeneration. It preserves musculature attachments for the paraspinal muscles and therefore preserves the posterior tension band, leading to decreased risk of postoperative kyphosis, and has fewer complications and better overall patient reported outcomes. The concept has also been raised that because the lamina is elevated en bloc, the risk of neurologic injury is decreased because violation of the spinal canal with instrumentation is avoided, especially in the setting of severe stenosis.[44,45]

Currently, there are 3 techniques that have been described when performing expansile laminoplasties: (1) open-door laminoplasty, (2) sagittal spinous process-splitting technique, and (3) the expansive midline threadwire saw (T-saw) technique, which is a modification of the sagital spinous process-splitting technique.

The open-door technique was initially described in Japanese by Hirabayashi in 1978 and later described in English by Hirabayashi in 1983.[46] This technique is technically demanding and requires performing a bicortical unilateral trough laminectomy followed by a unicortical trough laminectomy on the contralateral side. In so doing, the bicortical trough is opened and hinges on the unicortical trough, allowing for an increased spinal canal diameter. The lamina is then held open with

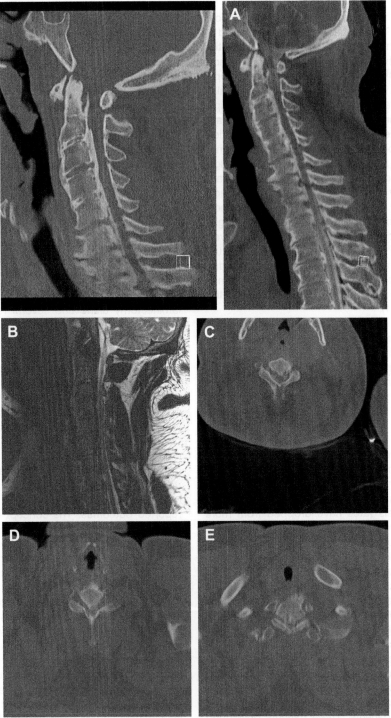

Fig. 1. Sagittal CT image of a 31-year-old man of Polynesian descent, presenting with a 6-month history of worsening gait, balance, and fine motor skills and complaining of pain and paresthesias in the bilateral C5, C6, and C7 dermatomes. Grossly myelopathic on examination with intact strength with muscle isolation. (*A*) Sagittal CT myelogram demonstrating OPLL, severe spinal canal stenosis from C2-3 to T1-T2, and autofusion from C2-5. (*B*) Sagittal T2-weighted MRI confirming severe spinal canal stenosis from C2-3 to T1-T2. (*C*) Axial CT myelogram at C2-3 disk space, portraying OPLL and spinal fluid circumferentially around spinal cord. (*D*) Axial CT myelogram at C6-7 disk space portraying near-complete loss of spinal fluid and deformation of the spinal cord secondary to OPLL. (*E*) Axial CT myelogram at T1-2 with reconstitution of spinal fluid and morphology of the cord. (*F–H*) Patient underwent C2-T2 posterior decompression with laminectomy and bilateral foraminotomy of the C5, C6, and C7 nerve roots and instrumented fusion from C3-T2 with C3-6 lateral mass screws and T1 and, T2 pedicle screws.

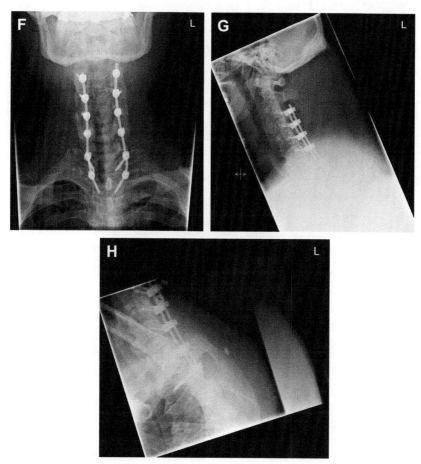

Fig. 1. (*continued*)

a cortical bone graft spacer with or without specially designed laminoplasty plates (**Fig. 2**).

The sagittal spinous process-splitting (French-door) technique was described by Kurokawa and colleagues in 1982 and published by Hoshi and collegues in 1996.[47] In this technique a high speed-burr was used to develop a sagittal split in the spinous process creating 2 hemilamina. Bilateral unicortical troughs are then developed at the edge of the lamina-lateral mass border and then the hemilamina are separated, like the opening of a French door, and held open with cortical bone grafts that are secured with wire to the lamina. This technique is also effective at expanding the spinal canal. This technique has several theoretic advantages over the open-door technique: (1) the posterior arch can be symmetrically reconstructed, (2) the expanded spinal canal is safely held open with cortical bone grafts with a safer distance from the spinal cord, and (3) the lateral epidural vein plexus is avoided. The main disadvantage, and likely the reason for its limited use,

is the danger of spinal cord injury during the sagittal splitting with the high-speed burr.

The third technique is a modification of the sagittal spinous process-splitting technique described by Tomita and colleagues[43] and is called the expansive midline T-saw technique. This technique uses the same concept as the sagittal-split technique but instead of using a high-speed burr to split the spinous process, a T-saw is used. This technique theoretically improves the sagittal-split technique by sparing critical surfaces of bone that are crucial for expanding the spinal canal that the high-speed burr sacrifices. The expanded spinal canal is then held open with cortical grafts that are secured in place by wire through the lamina.

Many investigators have attempted to decipher the differences between laminoplasty and laminectomy and fusion in an attempt to define an optimal treatment. Heller and colleagues[48] retrospectively reviewed a matched cohort of 13 patients undergoing laminectomy and fusion and 13 patients

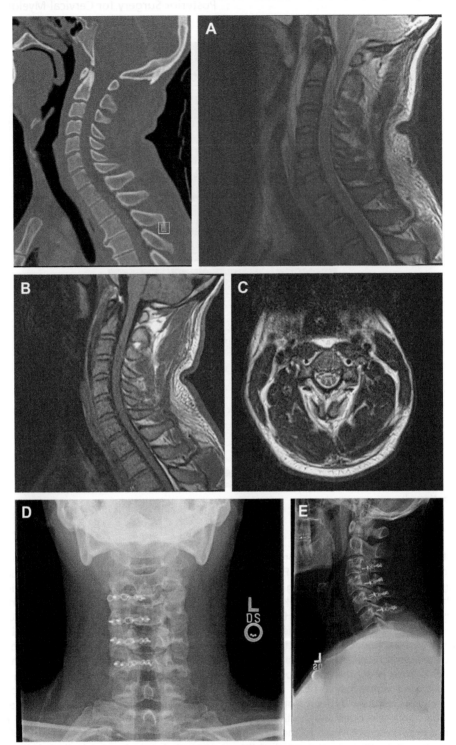

Fig. 2. 33-year-old man presented with acute central cord syndrome after performing back flips at a gym. Sagittal CT scan portrays normal cervical lordosis, minimal evidence of spondylosis, and no fractures noted on CT scan. Pavlov ratio is noted in **Fig. 1**. Pavlov's ratio at the C4 vertebral body measures 0.62. (*A, B*) Sagittal T1-weighted and T2-weighted MRI portraying congenital stenosis with cord signal change from C2-4 representing ischemia, edema, and microhemorrhage within the cord. (*C*) Axial T2-weighted MRI confirming intramedullary cord signal change at C3. (*D, E*) Patient underwent open-door laminoplasty at C3, C4, C5, and C6 with partial laminectomy of C2 and C7 using allograft cortical bone and specially designed laminoplasty plates (Synthes, Paoli, Pennsylvania). (*F*) Pavlov's ratio at the C4 vertebral body measures 0.92 postoperative T2-weighted sagittal MRI portraying maturation of cord injury and expanded spinal canal. (*G*) Postoperative sagittal CT scan portraying improved spinal canal dimensions, with Pavlov ratio. Postoperative canal. (*H*) Postoperative axial CT of C4 portraying the laminoplasty technique with a unicortical trough and an interposition cortical graft and plate.

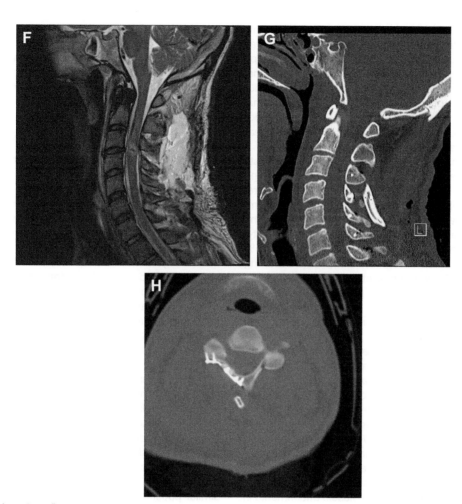

Fig. 2. (*continued*)

undergoing laminoplasty. With a mean follow-up of 26 months, they found greater improvement in the laminoplasty group than the fusion group with both objective findings (Nurick scores) and subjective findings (strength, dexterity, sensation, and gait). They also reported no complications in the laminoplasty group and 14 complications in 9 patients in the laminectomy and fusion group (worsening myelopathy, increased kyphosis, nonunion, instrumentation failure, persistent graft site harvest pain, subjacent degeneration requiring reoperation, and deep infection). They concluded that laminoplasty may be preferable to laminectomy and fusion in the treatment of multilevel cervical myelopathy.

In a larger retrospective matched cohort study of 121 patients from 2002 to 2007, Woods and colleagues[49] reported on 82 patients who underwent laminectomy and fusion and 39 who underwent laminoplasty, with an average follow-up of 24 months. Reviewing alignment changes, there was a significant difference from preoperative to

postopoperative in the 2 groups, with 2.57° loss of lordosis in the laminectomy and fusion group and 0.57° in the laminoplasty group, although this is not likely clinically significant. Patient-reported outcomes were similar between the 2 groups, as were the complication rates, with 2% and 5% requiring reoperation in the laminoplasty and laminectomy/fusion groups, respectively. The investigators concluded that prospective randomized trials are needed to determine if one procedure is truly superior.

Recently, a small prospective randomized trial was performed by Manzano and colleagues.[50] They randomized 16 patients to laminectomy and fusion or laminoplasty between 2006 and 2008 with 1-year follow-up data, including Short Form-36, Neck Disability Index, Nurick, and mJOA scores. They reported similar outcome measures in each group but the laminoplasty group had significantly improved Nurick scores at 1 year. The laminectomy and fusion group had a 75% decrease in cervical range of motion between C2 and C7 whereas the laminoplasty group had only a 20% decline. They also evaluated the overall increase in canal diameter between the 2 groups at 1 year and noted a significant increase in canal diameter in the laminectomy and fusion group, but they also noted a suggestion of decreased canal diameter of the adjacent level in the laminectomy and fusion group in as little as 1 year postoperatively.

The risks and complications of laminoplasty have been discussed in detail by Ratliff and Cooper[51] in their metanalysis of the literature. Loss of alignment, loss of motion, and long-term postoperative neck pain seem to be among the most common complications of laminoplasty. Loss of alignment occurs in approximately 35% of patients, with progressive kyphosis occurring in 10%. Cervical range of motion decreases by 15% to 50%. Axial neck pain after laminoplasty is even more common, ranging from 25% to 60% in the literature. It seems to vary with the laminoplasty technique.

Many investigators believe that preservation of the C2 and C7 muscle attachments decreases neck pain after laminoplasty. Hosono and colleagues[52] showed that avoiding dissection of the C7 muscle attachments by stopping the laminoplasty at C6 significantly decreased postoperative neck pain (5.4% vs 29%; $P = .015$). Sakaura and colleagues[53] discussed maintaining the muscular attachments at C2 and C7 as a way to limit postoperative neck pain and showed that patients with or without preservation of the muscle attachments in the intermediate cervical spine (C3 through 6) had no difference in pain as long as the superior and inferior attachments were maintained. The incidence of postoperative neck pain at long-term follow-up in their group was only 11%.

The other complication worth discussing, although also seen in laminectomy and laminectomy and fusion patients, is C5 root palsy. The incidence seems consistent in reports at approximately 8%, with most being transient.[51] Satomi[54] reported a 7.8% incidence of arm weakness in 206 patients undergoing open-door laminoplasty. It has been suggested that posterior migration of the spinal cord with root stretch may be the cause of this complication, although some investigators refute this. Hatta and colleagues[55] showed that by performing selective laminoplasty they were able to limit posterior migration of the spinal cord from an average 2.7 mm to 1.1 mm, likewise dropping the incidence from 8% (as in previous studies) to 0%. This was not a significant difference due to low numbers in the study groups; an analysis of the 2 patients who developed the C5 palsy showed that one had posterior cord migration of

3.1 mm whereas the other had only 0.1 mm of migration.

Laminoplasty is a safe and efficacious way to treat patients with CSM. It allows for decompression of the spinal cord without fusion while maintaining stability and some motion.

SUMMARY

Because of the lack of well-designed prospective randomized studies in patients with CSM it remains unclear as to the optimal treatment regimen and optimal timing of treatment. What is known is that patients with severe myelopathy report improved outcomes and improved neurologic recovery after surgical decompression. In the setting of multilevel spondylotic myelopathy with preserved cervical sagittal alignment, the posterior approach is favored. In most centers, decompressive laminectomy alone has been largely abandoned due to late neurologic decline and progressive kyphotic deformity. Because of improved patient outcome data, decreased complication rates, and improved neurologic recovery rates on instrumented posterior decompressions (fusion or laminoplasty), these techniques are preferred. Variables to consider when deciding between laminectomy and fusion versus laminoplasty include preoperative axial neck pain scores, cervical sagittal alignment, the degree of stenosis, and the absence or presence of pre-existing ankylosis because both of these techniques have similar patient outcome scores and complication profiles.

REFERENCES

1. Rao R. Neck pain, cervical radiculopathy, and cervical myelopathy: pathophysiology, natural history, and clinical evaluation. J Bone Joint Surg Am 2002; 84(10):1872–81.
2. Sampath P, Bendebba M, Davis JD, et al. Outcome of patients treated for cervical myelopathy. A prospective, multicenter study with independent clinical review. Spine (Phila Pa 1976) 2000;25(6):670–6.
3. Kadanka Z, Mares M, Bednanik J, et al. Approaches to spondylotic cervical myelopathy: conservative versus surgical results in a 3-year follow-up study. Spine (Phila Pa 1976) 2002;27(20):2205–10 [discussion: 2210–1].
4. Matz PG, Anderson PA, Holly LT, et al. The natural history of cervical spondylotic myelopathy. J Neurosurg Spine 2009;11(2):104–11.
5. Holly LT, Matz PG, Anderson PA, et al. Clinical prognostic indicators of surgical outcome in cervical spondylotic myelopathy. J Neurosurg Spine 2009; 11(2):112–8.

6. Imai T. Cervical spondylotic myelopathy and the antero-posterior diameter of the cervical canal. Nihon Seikeigeka Gakkai Zasshi 1970;44(6):429–38 [in Japanese].

7. White AA 3rd, Panjabi MM. Biomechanical considerations in the surgical management of cervical spondylotic myelopathy. Spine (Phila Pa 1976) 1988; 13(7):856–60.

8. Breig A, Turnbull I, Hassler O. Effects of mechanical stresses on the spinal cord in cervical spondylosis. A study on fresh cadaver material. J Neurosurg 1966;25(1):45–56.

9. Barnes MP, Saunders M. The effect of cervical mobility on the natural history of cervical spondylotic myelopathy. J Neurol Neurosurg Psychiatry 1984; 47(1):17–20.

10. Mair WG, Druckman R. The pathology of spinal cord lesions and their relation to the clinical features in protrusion of cervical intervertebral discs; a report of four cases. Brain 1953;76(1):70–91.

11. Ono K, Ebara S, Fuji T, et al. Myelopathy hand. New clinical signs of cervical cord damage. J Bone Joint Surg Br 1987;69(2):215–9.

12. Teresi LM, Lufkin RB, Reicher MA, et al. Asymptomatic degenerative disk disease and spondylosis of the cervical spine: MR imaging. Radiology 1987; 164(1):83–8.

13. Ohshio I, Hatayama A, Kaneda K, et al. Correlation between histopathologic features and magnetic resonance images of spinal cord lesions. Spine (Phila Pa 1976) 1993;18(9):1140–9.

14. Matsuda Y, Miyazaki K, Tada K, et al. Increased MR signal intensity due to cervical myelopathy. Analysis of 29 surgical cases. J Neurosurg 1991;74(6):887–92.

15. Shimomura T, Sumi M, Nishida K, et al. Prognostic factors for deterioration of patients with cervical spondylotic myelopathy after nonsurgical treatment. Spine (Phila Pa 1976) 2007;32(22):2474–9.

16. Spiker WR, Jeong EK, Daubs MD, et al. High resolution diffusion tensor imaging in cervical spondylotic myelopathy. Cervical Spine Research Society, 38th Annual Meeting. Charlotte (NC), December 2, 2010.

17. Shafaie FF, Wippold FJ 2nd, Gado M, et al. Comparison of computed tomography myelography and magnetic resonance imaging in the evaluation of cervical spondylotic myelopathy and radiculopathy. Spine (Phila Pa 1976) 1999;24(17):1781–5.

18. Iwasaki M, Okuda S, Miyauchi A, et al. Surgical strategy for cervical myelopathy due to ossification of the posterior longitudinal ligament: part 2: advantages of anterior decompression and fusion over laminoplasty. Spine (Phila Pa 1976) 2007;32(6): 654–60.

19. Edwards CC 2nd, Heller JG, Murakami H. Corpectomy versus laminoplasty for multilevel cervical myelopathy: an independent matched-cohort analysis. Spine (Phila Pa 1976) 2002;27(11):1168–75.

20. Yonenobu K, Hosono N, Iwasaki M, et al. Laminoplasty versus subtotal corpectomy. A comparative study of results in multisegmental cervical spondylotic myelopathy. Spine (Phila Pa 1976) 1992; 17(11):1281–4.

21. Sodeyama T, Goto S, Mochizuki M, et al. Effect of decompression enlargement laminoplasty for posterior shifting of the spinal cord. Spine (Phila Pa 1976) 1999;24(15):1527–31 [discussion: 1531–2].

22. Arnold H, Feldmann U, Missler U. Chronic spondylogenic cervical myelopathy. A critical evaluation of surgical treatment after early and long-term follow-up. Neurosurg Rev 1993;16(2):105–9.

23. Bishara SN. The posterior operation in treatment of cervical spondylosis with myelopathy: a long-term follow-up study. J Neurol Neurosurg Psychiatry 1971;34(4):393–8.

24. Carol MP, Ducker TB. Cervical spondylitic myelopathies: surgical treatment. J Spinal Disord 1988;1(1): 59–65.

25. Kato Y, Iwasaki M, Fuji T, et al. Long-term follow-up results of laminectomy for cervical myelopathy caused by ossification of the posterior longitudinal ligament. J Neurosurg 1998;89(2):217–23.

26. Matsunaga S, Sakou T, Nakanisi K. Analysis of the cervical spine alignment following laminoplasty and laminectomy. Spinal Cord 1999;37(1):20–4.

27. Perez-Lopez C, Isla A, Alvarez F, et al. Efficacy of arthrodesis in the posterior approach of cervical myelopathy: comparative study of a series of 36 cases. Neurocirugia (Astur) 2001;12(4):316–23 [discussion: 323–4, in Spanish].

28. Hamanishi C, Tanaka S. Bilateral multilevel laminectomy with or without posterolateral fusion for cervical spondylotic myelopathy: relationship to type of onset and time until operation. J Neurosurg 1996;85(3): 447–51.

29. Herkowitz HN. A comparison of anterior cervical fusion, cervical laminectomy, and cervical laminoplasty for the surgical management of multiple level spondylotic radiculopathy. Spine 1988;13(7): 774–80.

30. Halvorsen CM, Lied B, Harr ME, et al. Surgical mortality and complications leading to reoperation in 318 consecutive posterior decompressions for cervical spondylotic myelopathy. Acta Neurol Scand 2011;123:358–65.

31. Wimmer C, Gluch H, Franzreb M, et al. Predisposing factors for infection in spine surgery: a survey of 850 spinal procedures. J Spinal Disord 1998;11(2):124–8.

32. Yukawa Y, Kato F, Ito K, et al. Laminoplasty and skip laminectomy for cervical compressive myelopathy: range of motion, postoperative neck pain, and surgical outcomes in a randomized prospective study. Spine 2007;32:1980–5.

33. Callahan RA, Johnson RM, Margolis RN, et al. Cervical facet fusion for control of instability

following laminectomy. J Bone Joint Surg Am 1977;
59(8):991–1002.

34. Roy-Camille R, Saillant G. Surgery of the cervical spine. 3. Complex fractures of the lower cervical spine. Tetraplegia. Nouv Presse Med 1972;1(40):2707–9 [in French].

35. Magerl F, Seeman PS, Grob D. Stable dorsal fusion of cervical spine (C2–T1) using hook plates. The Cervical Spine 1. New York: Springer Verlag; 1987.

36. Heller JG, Carlson GD, Abitbol JJ, et al. Anatomic comparison of the Roy-Camille and Magerl techniques for screw placement in the lower cervical spine. Spine (Phila Pa 1976) 1991;16(Suppl 10):S552–7.

37. Barrey C, Mertens P, Jund J, et al. Quantitative anatomic evaluation of cervical lateral mass fixation with a comparison of the Roy-Camille and the Magerl screw techniques. Spine (Phila Pa 1976) 2005;30(6):E140–7.

38. Rihn JA, Lawrence J, Gates C, et al. Adjacent segment disease after cervical spine fusion. Instr Course Lect 2009;58:747–56.

39. Miyazaki K, Tada K, Matsuda Y, et al. Posterior extensive simultaneous multisegment decompression with posterolateral fusion for cervical myelopathy with cervical instability and kyphotic and/or S-shaped deformities. Spine (Phila Pa 1976) 1989;14(11):1160–70.

40. Katonis P, Papadakis SA, Galanakos S, et al. Lateral mass screw complications: analysis of 1662 screws. J Spinal Disord Tech 2011;24(7):415–20.

41. Hilibrand AS, Carlson GD, Palumbo MA, et al. Radiculopathy and myelopathy at segments adjacent to the site of a previous anterior cervical arthrodesis. J Bone Joint Surg Am 1999;81(4):519–28.

42. Graham AW, Swank ML, Kinard RE, et al. Posterior cervical arthrodesis and stabilization with a lateral mass plate. Clinical and computed tomographic evaluation of lateral mass screw placement and associated complications. Spine (Phila Pa 1976) 1996;21(3):323–8 [discussion: 329].

43. Tomita K, Kawahara N, Toribatake Y, et al. Expansive midline T-saw laminoplasty (modified spinous process-splitting) for the management of cervical myelopathy. Spine (Phila Pa 1976) 1998;23(1):32–7.

44. Lee TT, Manzano GR, Green BA. Modified open-door cervical expansive laminoplasty for spondylotic myelopathy: operative technique, outcome, and predictors for gait improvement. J Neurosurg 1997;86(1):64–8.

45. Satomi K, Nishu Y, Kohno T, et al. Long-term follow-up studies of open-door expansive laminoplasty for cervical stenotic myelopathy. Spine (Phila Pa 1976) 1994;19(5):507–10.

46. Hirabayashi K, Watanabe K, Wakano K, et al. Expansive open-door laminoplasty for cervical spinal stenotic myelopathy. Spine (Phila Pa 1976) 1983;8(7):693–9.

47. Hoshi K, Kurokawa T, Nakamura K, et al. Expansive cervical laminoplasties–observations on comparative changes in spinous process lengths following longitudinal laminal divisions using autogenous bone or hydroxyapatite spacers. Spinal Cord 1996;34(12):725–8.

48. Heller JG, Edwards CC 2nd, Murakami H, et al. Laminoplasty versus laminectomy and fusion for multilevel cervical myelopathy: an independent matched cohort analysis. Spine (Phila Pa 1976) 2001;26(12):1330–6.

49. Woods BI, Hohl J, Lee J, et al. Laminoplasty versus laminectomy and fusion for multilevel cervical spondylotic myelopathy. Clin Orthop Relat Res 2011;469(3):688–95.

50. Manzano GR, Casella G, Wang MY, et al. A prospective, randomized trial comparing expansile cervical laminoplasty versus cervical laminectomy and fusion for multi-level cervical myelopathy. Neurosurgery 2011. [Epub ahead of print].

51. Ratliff JK, Cooper PR. Cervical laminoplasty: a critical review. J Neurosurg 2003;98(Suppl 3):230–8.

52. Hosono N, Sakaura H, Mukai Y, et al. C3-6 laminoplasty takes over C3-7 laminoplasty with significantly lower incidence of axial neck pain. Eur Spine J 2006;15(9):1375–9.

53. Sakaura H, Hosono N, Mukai Y, et al. Preservation of muscles attached to the C2 and C7 spinous processes rather than subaxial deep extensors reduces adverse effects after cervical laminoplasty. Spine (Phila Pa 1976) 2010;35(16):E782–6.

54. Satomi K, Ogawa J, Ishii Y, et al. Short-term complications and long-term results of expansive open-door laminoplasty for cervical stenotic myelopathy. Spine J 2001;1(1):26–30.

55. Hatta Y, Shiraishi T, Hase H, et al. Is posterior spinal cord shifting by extensive posterior decompression clinically significant for multisegmental cervical spondylotic myelopathy? Spine (Phila Pa 1976) 2005;30(21):2414–9.

Anterior Approach for Complex Cervical Spondylotic Myelopathy

Krzysztof B. Siemionow, MD[a],*, Sergey Neckrysh, MD[b]

KEYWORDS

- Cervical spondylotic myelopathy • Degeneration
- Cervical spondylosis
- Ossification of posterior longitudinal ligament

Cervical spondylotic myelopathy (CSM) is a slowly progressive process that can be summarized as a gradual, progressive worsening of symptoms and a decline in functional status. In 1952, Brain and colleagues[1] reported the first large series of patients with CSM. CSM is a result of the reduction in the effective space available for the spinal cord. The resultant changes in the spinal segments may compromise the integrity of the spinal cord secondary to static, dynamic, or ischemic mechanisms.[2,3] CSM is the most common type of spinal cord dysfunction affecting individuals more than 55 years of age.[3,4] Surgical treatment remains the most reliable and predictable method of preventing further neurologic deterioration.

SURGICAL RATIONALE AND DECISION MAKING

The primary treatment of patients diagnosed with CSM is surgical. Nonoperative treatment consisting of medication, traction, or cervical collars has not been shown to alter the natural course of the disease.[5] Up to 50% of patients treated conservatively deteriorate neurologically over time.[6–9] Clarke and Robinson[6] reported that 5% of patients deteriorate quickly, 20% have a gradual but steady decline in function, and 70% have

a stepwise progression in their symptoms. Surgical intervention within 1 year of onset of symptoms can alter the natural history and change the prognosis of patients with CSM.[10–12]

There are multiple surgical approaches to treating patients with CSM. The primary goal of surgery is to increase the canal diameter and thus to decrease the risk of both static and dynamic compression. This approach arrests progression, and, if done early enough in the disease process, can improve neurologic function. There are multiple factors that must be taken into account when considering either anterior or posterior decompression.[13]

APPLIED SURGICAL ANATOMY

Choice of approach is dictated by the location of the disorder. The sternocleidomastoid (SCM), the carotid sheath, and the longus coli muscle serve as landmarks that differentiate the various approaches to the cervical spine. For example, approach can be either medial or lateral to the sternocleidomastoid. The key to the anterior cervical approach is in understanding the relationship between the neural structures, the vascular structures, the musculovisceral column and the 3 layers of the cervical fascia (**Fig. 1**).

[a] Department of Orthopaedic Surgery, University of Illinois, 835 South Wolcott Avenue, Room E-270, Chicago, IL 60612, USA
[b] Department of Neurosurgery, University of Illinois, 835 South Wolcott Avenue, Room E-270, Chicago, IL 60612, USA
* Corresponding author.
E-mail address: siemiok@gmail.com

Orthop Clin N Am 43 (2012) 41–52
doi:10.1016/j.ocl.2011.09.002
0030-5898/12/$ – see front matter © 2012 Elsevier Inc. All rights reserved.

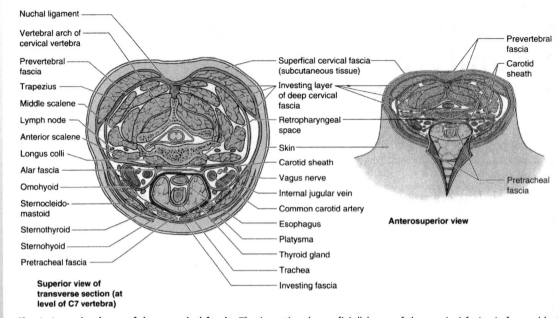

Fig. 1. Investing layer of deep cervical fascia: The investing (superficial) layer of the cervical fasica is formed by the investing layer of deep cervical fascia. The platysma and the external jugular vein are the only structures superficial to it. The superficial layer surrounds the neck circumferentially and invests the sternocleidomastoid and the trapezius. Opening the superficial layer of the cervical fascia is a critical first step in any anterior cervical approach. **Pretracheal layer of deep cervical fascia**: The thin pretracheal (visceral) layer is limited to the anterior part of the neck. The visceral layer encloses the trachea, the esophagus, and the thyroid gland. The pretracheal fascia blends laterally with the carotid sheath and must be separated at the medial border of the carotid sheath to gain entrance to the retropharyngeal space. The superior and inferior thyroid vessels run from the carotid sheath through the pretracheal fascia to the midline and may need to be ligated. **Prevertebral fascia**: The last fascial layer lines is the prevertebral layer. It covers the anterior aspect of the anterior longitudinal ligament and the prevertebral muscles. (*From* Moore K, Dalley A. Clinically oriented anatomy. 4th edition. Lippincott Williams & Wilkins; 1999. p. 999. Figure 8.4; with permission.)

AT-RISK STRUCTURES
Cervical Sympathetic Chain

The cervical sympathetic chain is located postero-medial to the carotid sheath and runs over the longus muscles.[14] It extends longitudinally from longus capitis to longus colli over the muscles and under the prevertebral fascia. From superior to inferior, longus colli muscle diverges laterally, whereas the cervical sympathetic chain converges medially at C6. The average distance between the cervical sympathetic chain and medial border of the longus colli muscle at C6 is 11.6 ($\pm$1.6) mm. The superior ganglion of the cervical sympathetic chain in all dissections was located at the level of the C4 vertebra.

Vertebral Artery

The vertebral artery originates from the subclavian or innominate artery and enters the transverse foramen (TF) of the sixth cervical vertebrae.[15,16] Before this, it is anterior to the transverse foraminae of C7. The artery passes through a series of foraminae until it

reaches the base of the axis. It then turns posteriorly to enter the foramen transversarium in the postero-lateral part of the ring of atlas and perforates the posterior atlantoaxial membrane to enter the foramen magnum. It then joins the contralateral vertebral artery to form the basilar artery, which supplies the brain stem and cerebellum.

The vertebral artery is intimately associated with the lateral border of the uncovertebral joint. Pait and colleagues[17] reported that the distance from the tip of the uncinate process to the verte-bral artery averaged 0.8 mm at C2 to C3 and 1.6 mm at C4 to C5. In a magnetic resonance imaging (MRI) study, Eskander and colleagues[18] reported that the smallest distance between the uncovertebral joint (measured from the medial aspect of the uncovertebral joint to the medial aspect of the vertebral artery) was 4.15 mm at C3. Caution should be exercised when the uncinate process is removed in an attempt to remove osteophytes. In a review of 10 cases of vertebral artery injury, Smith and colleagues[19] found that the use of a high-powered drill laterally was the most frequent cause of arterial injury. The surgeon must always check preoperative imaging for vertebral artery anomalies. There are 3 types of vertebral artery anomalies: (1) intraforaminal anomalies, (2) extraforaminal anomalies, and (3) arterial anomalies.[18]

Recurrent Laryngeal Nerve

Injury to the recurrent laryngeal nerve (RLN) is a commonly reported complication following anterior cervical spine surgery. The RLN innervates all the intrinsic muscles of the neck with the exception of the cricothyroid.[20] Almost all RLN injuries resolve over time; however, permanent paralysis rates have been reported in up to 3.5% of patients.[21,22] Several causes for RLN injury have been suggested, including postoperative edema, stretch-induced neuropraxia, direct nerve ligature, direct retractor-induced nerve trauma, and nerve impingement between the endotracheal tube and retractor.[23–25]

The right RLN branches from the vagus nerve at the level of T1 to T2. After looping around the subclavian artery, the right RLN becomes invested in the tracheoesophageal fascia (TEF). The RLN then travels superiorly and slightly anterior to the tracheoesophageal groove (TEG), before coursing between the trachea and the thyroid. In 82% (9 of 11) of right-sided dissections, the RLN entered the larynx at or inferior to C6 to C7.[26] After looping around the aortic arch, the left RLN becomes invested in the TEF inferior to the T2 level. The nerve then travels slightly anterior to the TEG and within the TEF before coursing between the trachea and thyroid. In all the left-sided dissections, the RLN entered the larynx at or inferior to C6 to C7.[26] The investigators concluded that both the left and the right RLNs had similar anatomic courses and received similar protection via surrounding soft tissue structures. From an anatomic perspective, the investigators did not appreciate a side-to-side difference superior to this level that could place either nerve at greater risk for injury.

Carotid Sheath

The carotid sheath contains the common and internal carotid arteries, the internal jugular vein, the vagus nerve, deep cervical lymph nodes, carotid sinus nerve, and sympathetic nerve fibers. The carotid sheath is a fascial investment that blends anteriorly with the investing and pretracheal layers of fascia. During surgical dissection, the carotid sheath is protected by the anterior border of the SCM. Care must be taken when placing and removing retractors to avoid vascular injury.

Esophagus

The esophagus is a thin ribbonlike structure that is located anterior to the retropharyngeal space. To prevent injury, it is critical to identify the esophagus during the approach. Placing an orogastric tube preoperatively can aide in esophageal identification.

SURGICAL CONSIDERATIONS
Sagittal Alignment

Cervical sagittal alignment is an important consideration, because it affects the surgical treatment options and approach. The normal range of cervical lordosis is 40° (±9.7°) with most occurring between C1 and C2 while the occipital cervical junction is in kyphosis.[27] The average lordosis between C4 and C7 is 6°, making this one of the flatter parts of the cervical spine. The presence of a cervical kyphosis poses a challenge for posteriorly based procedures. Because cervical laminectomy or laminoplasty are dependant on the posterior drift of the spinal cord, they are less effective in the kyphotic spine.

Restoring sagittal alignment should also be one of the goals of surgery and this may be more difficult to achieve from a posterior-only approach. Some of these difficulties may be overcome with an anterior approach or a combination anterior-posterior approach.

Disease Type and Location

The type and location of spinal cord compression dictate the surgical approach. The compression can be either soft or hard. Soft compression results from noncalcified soft tissues, whereas calcified or hard compressive disorders need to be identified because their presence may alter the surgical approach used to achieve decompression. Ventrally located compressive disorders can be localized to the level of the disk, dorsal to the vertebral body, or both. It can involve 1 or multiple levels. The addition of a dorsally located compressive disorder increases the complexity of decision making. Simple ventrally localized degenerative changes, such as anterior osteophytes or disk herniations, should be approached anteriorly to ensure adequate decompression. Dorsal compression, such as from ligamentum flavum hypertrophy or multilevel ossification of the posterior longitudinal ligament, should be approached posteriorly to achieve direct cord decompression. Sagittal alignment needs to be verified with a standing lateral radiograph. Because dorsal compression tends to be more generalized than focal, a posterior approach can more easily decompress multiple levels than anterior decompression. Generally, 1-level to 3-level ventral compressive disorders can be addressed from an anterior-only approach, whereas 4-level disorders should be addressed from a posterior approach or a combination anterior-posterior approach (**Fig. 2**).[28]

Motion Preservation

The incidence of adjacent segment degeneration following anterior cervical fusion has been reported to be approximately 3% per year.[29] Motion preservation technology has gained popularity because it is intended to reduce abnormal stresses transferred to adjacent levels, thus theoretically reducing the chance of developing adjacent segment degeneration.[30–33] Clinically, the risk of developing adjacent segment degeneration has been shown to be equivalent to both fusion and arthroplasty.[34–36] There is also a concern that motion preservation may continue to result in microtrauma to the spinal cord, thus negatively affecting clinical outcomes. Buchowski and colleagues[37] reported that 2 years after surgery, cervical arthroplasty outcomes were equivalent to arthrodesis for the treatment of cervical myelopathy for a single-level abnormality localized to the disk space. Hybrid surgery in which 1 level is fused and the second level is treated with cervical arthroplasty has been reported to be superior to 2-level anterior cervical diskectomy and fusion (ACDF) in better Neck Disability Index recovery, lower postoperative

neck pain, faster C2 to C7 range of motion (ROM) recovery, and less adjacent ROM increase.[38,39] Cervical arthroplasty is an option for the treatment of uncomplicated CSM. Whether adjacent level degeneration is the result of the fusion, or simply the expression of the natural deterioration of the motion segments, is unclear.

SURGICAL OPTIONS
Corpectomy Versus ACDF for 2-Level Disease

When dealing with multilevel disease, the surgeon has to decide whether to perform an ACDF, a corpectomy, or a hybrid procedure (**Fig. 3**). Both have unique advantages and disadvantages. The location of the disorder plays a dominant role in the decision-making process. Compression localized to the level of the disk can be approached with either procedure, whereas a disorder localized dorsal to the vertebral body needs to be treated with a corpectomy. The main advantage of a corpectomy in treating a multilevel disorder is the decreased number of graft-bone surfaces that need to fuse. In a 2-level ACDF, there are 4 bone-graft interfaces, compared with only 2 for a corpectomy. The theoretic risk of pseudarthrosis is therefore generally less with corpectomy than with multilevel ACDF. In a recent meta-analysis Fraser and Härtl[40] reported that, for 2-disk–level disease, there was no significant difference between anterior cervical diskectomy with a plate system and corpectomy with a plate system. However, for 3-disk–level disease, the

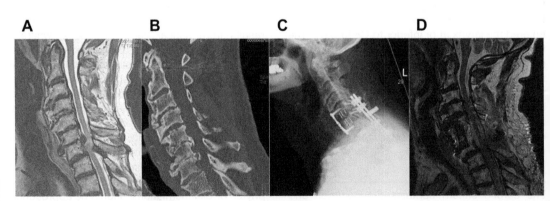

Fig. 2. (*A*) An 82 year-old diabetic male presented with painless progressive lower extremity weakness and long tract sings. His cervical T-2 weighted MRI was significant for spinal cord compression at C6-C7 with myelomalacia secondary to a large disc osteophyte complex; posterior ligamentum flavum buckling and spinal cord compression at C7-T1; Anterolisthesis of C7 on T1. (*B*) Sagittal CT scan demonstrates moderate disc calcification and osteophyte formation at C5-C6 and marked disc calcification and osteophyte formation at C6-C7. The patient has circumferential cervical spinal cord compression in addition to the C7-T1 anterolisthesis. This type of spinal cord compression would best be addressed with an anterior-posterior decompression and fusion. (*C*) Lateral x-ray demonstrating C6 corpectomy and anterior instrumented fusion from C5-C7 with posterior decompression of C7-T1 and posterior instrumented fusion from C5-T2. (*D*) Post decompression T-2 weighted MRI demonstrating a fully decompressed spinal cord.

A B C D

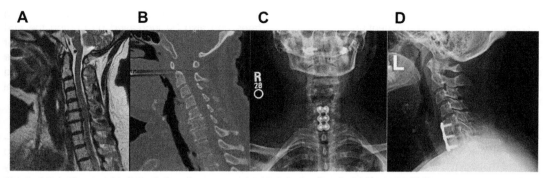

Fig. 3. (*A*) A 62 year-old diabetic female presented with burning hands and gait instability. T-2 weighted MRI of the cervical spine demonstrates spinal cord compression secondary to spondylosis at C5-C6 and C6-C7. (*B*) Sagittal CT scan demonstrates calcification of both the C5-C6 and C6-C7 discs. Both the MRI and the CT scan confirm that the compression is localized to the level of the disc space. This particular case can be treated with either a C6 corpectomy or a 2 level ACDF. (*C, D*) AP and Lateral post-operative x-rays demonstrate a 2 level ACDF with a semiconstrained cervical plate.

investigators reported that corpectomy with plate placement was associated with higher fusion rates than diskectomy with plate placement. Park and colleagues[41] compared 2-level diskectomy with single-level corpectomy and reported comparable results for sagittal alignment, cervical lordosis, graft subsidence, and adjacent level ossification. Wang and colleagues[42] compared 32 patients undergoing a 2-level ACDF with autograft with 20 patients with a 1-level corpectomy and anterior instrumentation. The investigators reported similar fusion and complication rates between the 2 groups. In contrast with these studies, Guo and colleagues[43] reported that ACDF was superior in most outcomes to anterior cervical corpectomy and fusion and anterior cervical hybrid decompression and fusion. The investigators concluded that, if the compressive disorder could be resolved by diskectomy, then an ACDF is the treatment of choice.

ACDF

ACDF is commonly used in the treatment of CSM. This approach allows for spinal cord and nerve root decompression secondary to herniated disks and spondylotic bone spurs.[44] With the use of an operating microscope, excellent visualization of the disk space, uncovertebral joints, and spinal cord is possible. A thorough diskectomy and meticulous end-plate preparation are critical for neural decompression, disk space distraction, and interbody fusion. This surgical approach uses intermuscular plane and is usually better tolerated than posterior surgery. Nerve root decompression can also be performed by resecting the uncovertebral spurs and foraminal decompression. Correction of sagittal plane deformities

can be achieved by using lordotic intervertebral spacers. In addition, restoring anterior disk height increases the foraminal space and indirectly decompresses the nerve root. Single-level ACDF is associated with high fusion rates, particularly when used in conjunction with anterior plating.[45,46] In a study of 2-level and 3-level ACDF with anterior plating, Samartidis and colleagues[47] reported a fusion rate of 97.5% with either autograft or allograft. Wang and colleagues[46] reported a high percentage of good to excellent clinical outcomes and a low incidence of segmental kyphosis and pseudarthrosis using anterior cervical plating.

Corpectomy

Cervical corpectomy is performed by removing the disk above and below the vertebral body to be resected. This removal is followed by resection of the vertebral body itself. Anterior osteophytes, ossification of the posterior longitudinal ligament (PLL), and disk herniations located behind the vertebral body can be addressed with this approach. Preoperative kyphosis can also be corrected. The procedure involves the creation of a trough in the middle portion of the vertebral body. It is critical to identify the lateral cortical wall of the vertebral body, which is located at the junction of the transverse process and the vertebral body. Identification of this landmark keeps the trough centered and symmetric, thereby avoiding injury to the vertebral artery. The wide trough permits extensive visualization of the disk, PLL, and osteophytes, thereby allowing a safe resection of all compressive disease. The strut graft for reconstruction following corpectomy is typically either structural iliac crest autograft, fibula allograft, or a cage construct packed with autograft.[48,49] The incidence of surgical-related complications was associated with increasing patient age.[50] Potential technical issues with these grafts include difficulty in restoring normal lordosis, graft dislodgment, graft migration, and, more commonly, graft subsidence.[51] Anterior cervical plating is recommended for cervical corpectomy.[48,52,53]

Multilevel Corpectomy

Multilevel disorder may require more complex surgical management. For corpectomy involving 3 or more levels, an anterior-posterior fusion has been recommended.[54–56] Stand-alone anterior constructs have a high rate of graft migration, dislodgment, and pseudarthrosis.[55,56] Construct motion has been shown to be lowest in a combined anterior-posterior instrumentation model.[57,58] Circumferential cervical fusion has been shown to maximize cervical stability and decrease the incidence of graft migration or dislodgment.[59] Accosta and colleagues[54] reported that multilevel instrumented corpectomy offered a biomechanically stable fixation and allowed for significant correction of preexisting kyphosis. Supplemental posterior instrumentation was thought to limit delayed cage subsidence and loss of sagittal balance after this procedure. In the absence of posterior instrumentation, a large moment arm is created with an anterior-only construct. This construct can lead to loss of stability and pistoning or toggling of the graft and its eventual dislodgment, even with the use of an anterior plate or supplemental external fixation in a halo device. Vaccaro and colleagues[56] treated 45 patients with 2-level or 3-level corpectomies and anterior plating. No supplemental posterior instrumentation was used. The investigators reported a 9% dislodgment rate in the 2-levelcorpectomy and 50% dislodgment rate in the 3-level corpectomy. Graft migration occurred despite the use of a halo in 10 of 12 patients who underwent a 3-level instrumented corpectomy. Sasso and colleagues[55] reported a 71% catastrophic failure rate involving graft-plate dislodgment that occurred within 2 months of instrumented 3-level corpectomy. An additional advantage of supplemental posterior instrumented fusion is the ability to perform a posterior laminectomy, if needed, to further decompress the neural elements.

TECHNICAL
Graft Choice: Allograft Versus Autograft

When cervical plating is used, using allograft versus autograft has not been shown to make a significant difference in the rate of pseudarthrosis with up to a 3-level ACDF.[45,47] A longer time to union was seen with allograft, although this difference was not clinically significant. Fusion rates can also be increased by burring the end plates down to bleeding bone to augment graft incorporation. This technique was shown to be associated with minimal graft subsidence and decreased the pseudarthrosis rate to approximately 4.4% per level.[60]

Anterior Cervical Plating

Anterior cervical plating has commonly been used to stabilize ACDF and corpectomies, and many studies have found a higher fusion rate with the use of a cervical plate.[1,2] Some of the other benefits of plating include improved initial stability; decreased need for orthotics; and reduction in complications from graft dislocation, end-plate fracture, and kyphotic collapse.[1,2] The original anterior cervical plate designs provided rigid fixation between segments, acting as a tension band system in extension and as a buttress plate in flexion. These plate types are commonly referred to as constrained devices. It is hypothesized that these rigid fixation devices are load bearing and may eliminate the mechanical loads on the bone graft, which are thought to be important for fusion. These static designs may also prevent any settling from occurring, thus leaving a gap between the bone graft and the end plate. To overcome these disadvantages, dynamic anterior cervical plates have been introduced that allow for graft loading by axial settling. In biomechanical cadaveric cervical corpectomy studies comparing dynamic and static plates, Brodke and colleagues[61,62] showed that more load sharing occurred in dynamic cervical plates, because these plate designs allowed for axial settling to make up for graft resorption during the postoperative period. In the experimental situation of a collapsed bone graft, less motion was found with dynamic plates. Fogel and colleagues[63] reported that the static plate had significantly higher graft loads in extension and significant loss of graft load in flexion, whereas the dynamic plate maintained a reasonable graft load throughout the ROM even when graft contact was imperfect. The design of the plate does not affect the outcomes in single-level fusions but statistics indicate that multiple-level fusions may have better clinical outcomes when a dynamic plate design is used.[64]

Anterior Cervical Plate Location and Adjacent Segment Degeneration

Cervical plate location has implications for developing adjacent level degeneration. Koller and colleagues[65] reported that progression of adjacent segment disease after instrumented ACDF was significantly linked to a plate to adjacent disk distance of less than 3 mm. Park and colleagues[66] recommended that anterior cervical plates be placed at least 5 mm away from the adjacent disk spaces to decrease the likelihood of moderate-to-severe adjacent level ossification. Based on their experience with static and dynamic anterior cervical plating, DuBois and colleagues[67] suggested that placing instrumentation at least 3 mm from the adjacent level disk would decrease the potential for adjacent level changes. These studies suggest that extension of plates toward adjacent healthy disks, and perhaps extensive surgical dissection and damage to the anterior longitudinal ligament, are contributing factors in the development of adjacent segment disease.

Decompression

The causes of postoperative deterioration in function include spinal cord injury during surgery, malalignment of the spine associated with graft complication, and epidural hematoma.[68] The extent of spinal decompression remains controversial.[69,70] Removal of posterior osteophytes and resection of the PLL increase the space available for the spinal cord. However, this is more technically challenging, adds time to the procedure, and increases the risk of neural injury and postoperative epidural hematoma.[68,70] Recently, Wang and colleagues[71] reported that removal of PLL was generally safe, although more technically demanding. More importantly, the investigators reported a significant improvement in Japanese Orthopaedic Association (JOA) scores in patients in whom the PLL was resected.

It has been suggested that the posterior osteophytes resorb once the spine is fused and segmental motion is eliminated.[72] Stevens and colleagues[73] showed that there was no evidence of remodeling or resorption of osteophytes, and persistent osteophytes continued to deform the spinal cord for up to 12 years after fusion. This finding suggests that osteophyte removal should be performed whenever possible.

COMPLICATIONS

Anterior cervical procedures are successful in treating most patients with cervical myelopathy. Adverse events associated with anterior cervical procedures are listed in **Table 1**. Because most patients who undergo surgery for cervical myelopathy are elderly, their ability to tolerate complications is poor. Appropriate strategies must be used to prevent these complications, and the surgeon should have an understanding of how to

Table 1
Adverse events associated with anterior cervical spine surgery

Adverse Event	
Intraoperative	Reported Incidence (%)
Esophageal injury	0.2–0.4
Vertebral artery injury	0.3
Dural tear	3.7
Spinal cord	0.2–0.9
Peripheral nerve injury or radiculopathy	0.2–3.2
Immediate to early postoperative (within 1 week)	
Airway compromise caused by airway edema or hematoma	1.7–6.0
Epidural hematoma	0.2–1.9
Radiculopathy	1.3
Intermediate to longer term postoperative (1 to 6 weeks)	
Dysphagia	28–57
Dysphonia	2–30
Bone graft extrusion	6–71
Wound infection	0.2–1.6

Data from Daniels AH, Riew KD, Yoo JU, et al. Adverse events associated with anterior cervical spine surgery. J Am Acad Orthop Surg 2008;16:729–38. *Data from* Refs.[97–100]

recognize and manage such events when they do arise.

RLN

Beutler and colleagues[74] reported that the incidence of RLN symptoms after surgery was 2.7% (9 of 328). The incidence of RLN symptoms was 2.1% with anterior cervical diskectomy, 3.5% with corpectomy (5 of 141), 3% with instrumentation (8 of 237), and 9.5% with reoperative anterior surgery (2 of 21). There was a significant increase in the rate of injury with revision anterior surgeries. The investigators reported no association between the side of approach and the incidence of RLN symptoms. Kilburg and colleagues[75] did not report any difference in RLN injury in their retrospective study of 1-level and 2-level ACDF. These rates are in contrast with those reported by Jung and colleagues.[24] These investigators used laryngoscopy to assess the incidence of laryngeal nerve palsy. The overall incidence was 24.2%, with most patients being asymptomatic. In a follow-up nonrandomized prospective observational study, Jung and Schramm[25] reported that the left-sided approach reduced the incidence of postoperative and permanent RLN palsy (RLNP) significantly with endotracheal cuff pressure reduction (<20 mm Hg) decreasing the rate of RLNP even more. The investigators concluded that anterior cervical spine surgery should be performed with a left-sided approach and, if possible, with an additional reduction of the endotracheal cuff pressure while the retractors are inserted.

Dysphagia

Dysphagia is frequently observed after anterior cervical procedures. It can be a result of local swelling secondary to tissue manipulation and retraction as well as graft or instrumentation prominence. After having cervical spine surgery, 71% of patients reported dysphagia at 2 weeks' follow-up.[76] This incidence decreased to 8% at 12 weeks' follow-up. The investigators observed a correlation between operative time and the severity of postoperative dysphagia. The risk of dysphagia increases with number of surgical vertebral levels.[77] Patients reporting dysphagia at 3 months had a significantly higher self-reported disability and lower physical health status at subsequent assessments.[77] Dysphagia was noted to be more common in women than in men. It has been suggested that a smoother and lower profile plate might decrease the incidence of dysphagia.[78]

Radiculopathy

Radiculopathy of C5 after decompression and multilevel corpectomy was noted first in the English literature by Shinomiya and colleagues.[79] There are several proposed hypothesis for the cause of C5 palsy. Tsuzuki and colleagues[80,81] suggested that an extradural tethering effect was a potential mechanism leading to postoperative radiculopathy. Postoperative anterior shift of the spinal cord in the presence of dural adhesions is plausible hypothesis for C5 palsy in anterior corpectomy.[82] Ikenaga and colleagues[82] reported that the incidence of C5 palsy after cervical corpectomy and fusion for myelopathy was 3.1%. Cord compression at C3 to C4 and C4 to C5 was significantly more severe in patients with paralysis than in those without paralysis. Wada and colleagues[83] reported an incidence of 4.4% for a mean of 2.5 levels fused, whereas Hashimoto reported it to be 8.5%.[84] The risk of neural injury was greatest for patients with ossification of the PLL and may be related to the magnitude of preexisting cord compression.[82] C5 palsy correlated with the presence of high signal changes in the spinal cord.[84] The investigators concluded that preexisting asymptomatic damage of the anterior horn cells at the C3 to C4 and C4 to C5 levels might participate in the development of motor weakness in combination with the nerve root lesions. Patients with less than 2/5 weakness on manual strength testing had a worse prognosis.[84]

Esophagus

Esophageal injury is a rare but catastrophic complication of anterior cervical spine surgery.[85] Esophageal injury incidence based on overall occurrence was 0.1%.[86] Patients with no antecedent risk factors had an incidence of 0.03%.[86]

CLINICAL OUTCOMES

Clinical outcomes after anterior cervical procedures usually show some functional improvement. In a study by Chagas and colleagues,[87] the mean Nurick score improved from 2.97 to 2.1 after anterior decompression. Rajashekar and Kumar[88] reported that the mean Nurick score improved from 4.24 to 2.47 after corpectomy. Corpectomy has been shown to increase the modified JOA (mJOA) score and thus the quality of life and activities of daily living.[71,89] Chibbaro and colleagues[89] reported an improvement in mJOA score from 12.2 to 15, whereas Wang and colleagues[71] reported an improvement from 10.4 to 15.2.

Gok and colleagues[90] reported significant improvement in Nurick grade in 93% of patients who underwent anterior surgery for CSM for primarily ventral disease or loss of cervical lordosis. The investigators suggested adding supplemental posterior fixation and arthrodesis in patients who undergo multilevel ventral decompression. Chagas and colleagues[87] reported that 80.6% of patients were very satisfied or satisfied with the outcome and would decide again for the surgery (87%) if the results were previously known. Sorar and colleagues[91] reported that 85% of patients treated with an anterior decompression experienced a 50% or more recovery rate as calculated using the Hirabayashi formula. Sakai and colleagues[92] reported that the mean Japanese Orthopedic Association score and the recovery rate in the anterior decompression and fusion group were superior to those in the French-door laminoplasty group.

Surgery for CSM is associated with significant functional recovery, which seems to reach a plateau at 6 months after surgery.[93] Age is a potential predictor of complications after decompressive surgery for CSM.[93] Nagashima and colleagues[94] reported that elderly patients aged 80 years or older regained approximately 40% of their function after surgery, and the incidence of postoperative complication was similar to that in younger patients.

Patients with an increase spinal cord intensity on T-2 weighted images usually had a low preoperative JOA score and experienced less improvement in neurologic function after surgery.[95] High intramedullary signal intensity change is a poor prognostic factor and the intramedullary contrast (gadolinium-diethylenetriaminepentaacetic acid [Gd-DTPA]) enhancement on preoperative MRI should be viewed as the worst predictor of surgical outcomes in cervical myelopathy.[96] Contrast (Gd-DTPA) enhancement and postoperative MRI are useful for identifying the prognosis of patients with poor neurologic recovery.

SUMMARY

CSM is a slowly progressive disease resulting from age-related degenerative changes in the spine that can lead to spinal cord dysfunction and significant functional disability. The degenerative changes and abnormal motion lead to vertebral body subluxation, osteophyte formation, ligamentum flavum hypertrophy, and spinal canal narrowing.

Repetitive movement during normal cervical motion may result in microtrauma to the spinal cord. Disease extent and location dictate the choice of surgical approach. Anterior spinal decompression and instrumented fusion is successful in preventing CSM progression and has been shown to result in functional improvement in most patients.

REFERENCES

1. Brain W, Northfield D, Wilkinson M. The neurological manifestations of cervical spondylosis. Brain 1952;75:187–225.
2. Fehlings M, Skaf G. A review of the pathophysiology of cervical spondylotic myelopathy with insights for potential novel mechanisms drawn from traumatic spinal cord injury. Spine 1998;23:2730–7.
3. Young W. Cervical spondylotic myelopathy: a common cause of spinal cord dysfunction in older persons. Am Fam Physician 2000;62:1064–70, 1073.
4. Bernhardt M, Hynes R, Blume H, et al. Cervical spondylotic myelopathy. J Bone Joint Surg Am 1993;75:119–28.
5. McCormick W, Steinmetz M, Benzel E. Cervical spondylotic myelopathy: make the difficult diagnosis then refer for surgery. Cleve Clin J Med 2003;70:10899–904.
6. Clarke E, Robinson P. Cervical myelopathy: a complication of cervical spondylosis. Brain 1956;79(3):483–510.
7. Epstein J. The surgical management of cervical spinal stenosis, spondylosis, and myeloradiculopathy by means of the posterior approach. Spine 1988;13(7):864–9.
8. Syman L, Lavender P. The surgical treatment of cervical spondylotic myelopathy. Neurology 1967; 17:117–26.
9. Roberts A. Myelopathy due to cervical spondylosis treated by collar immobilization. Neurology 1966; 16:951–4.
10. Montgomery D, Brower R. Cervical spondylotic myelopathy. Clinical syndrome and natural history. Orthop Clin North Am 1992;23(3):487–93.
11. Phillips D. Surgical treatment of myelopathy with cervical spondylosis. J Neurol Neurosurg Psychiatry 1973;36(5):879–84.
12. Ebersold M, Pare M, Quast L. Surgical treatment for cervical spondylotic myelopathy. J Neurosurg 1995;82(5):745–51.
13. Edwards CC 2nd, Riew K, Anderson P, et al. Cervical myelopathy: current diagnostic and treatment strategies. Spine J 2003;3:68–81.
14. Civelek E, Karasu A, Cansever T, et al. Surgical anatomy of the cervical sympathetic trunk during anterolateral approach to cervical spine. Eur Spine J 2008;17(8):991–5.
15. Lu J, Ebraheim N. The vertebral artery: surgical anatomy. Orthopedics 1999;22:1081–5.
16. Heary R, Todd A, Ludwig S. Surgical anatomy of the vertebral arteries. Spine 1996;21:2074–80.
17. Pait T, Killefer J, Arnautovic K. Surgical anatomy of the anterior cervical spine: the disc space, vertebral artery, and associated bony structures. Neurosurgery 1996;39(4):769–76.
18. Eskander M, Drew J, Aubin M, et al. Vertebral artery anatomy: a review of two hundred fifty magnetic resonance imaging scans. Spine (Phila Pa 1976) 2010;35(23):2035–40.
19. Smith M, Emery S, Dudley A. Vertebral artery injury during anterior decompression of the cervical spine. J Bone Joint Surg Br 1993;75:410–5.
20. Ebraheim N, Lu J, Skie M, et al. Vulnerability of the recurrent laryngeal nerve in the anterior approach to the lower cervical spine. Spine 1997;22(22):2664–7.
21. Apfelbaum R, Kriskovich M, Haller J. On the incidence, cause, and prevention of recurrent laryngeal nerve palsies during anterior cervical spine surgery. Spine 2000;25:2906–12.
22. Heeneman H. Vocal cord paralysis following approaches to the anterior cervical spine. Laryngoscope 1973;83:17–21.
23. Fountas K, Kapsalaki E, Nikolakakos L, et al. Anterior cervical discectomy and fusion associated complications. Spine 2007;32(21):2310–7.

24. Jung A, Schramm J, Lehnerdt K, et al. Recurrent laryngeal nerve palsy during anterior cervical spine surgery: a prospective study. J Neurosurg Spine 2005;2(2):123–7.

25. Jung A, Schramm J. How to reduce recurrent laryngeal nerve palsy in anterior cervical spine surgery: a prospective observational study. Neurosurgery 2010;67(1):10–5 [discussion: 15].

26. Haller J, Iwanik M, Shen F. Clinically relevant anatomy of recurrent laryngeal nerve. Spine (Phila Pa 1976) 2011. [Epub ahead of print].

27. Hardacker J, Shuford R, Capicotto R, et al. Radiographic standing cervical segmental alignment in adult volunteers without neck symptoms. Spine 1997;22:1472–80.

28. Herkowitz H, Kurz L, Overholt D. Surgical management of cervical soft disc herniation. A comparison between the anterior and posterior approach. Spine 1990;15(10):1026–30.

29. Hilibrand A, Carlson G, Palumbo M, et al. Radiculopathy and myelopathy at segments adjacent to the site of a previous anterior cervical arthrodesis. J Bone Joint Surg Am 1999;81(4):519–28.

30. Chang UK, Kim DH, Lee MC, et al. Changes in adjacent-level disc pressure and facet joint force after cervical arthroplasty compared with cervical discectomy and fusion. J Neurosurg Spine 2007;7(1):33–9.

31. Sasso RC, Best NM, Metcalf NH, et al. Motion analysis of Bryan cervical disc arthroplasty versus anterior discectomy and fusion: results from a prospective, randomized, multicenter, clinical trial. J Spinal Disord Tech 2008;21(6):393–9.

32. DiAngelo DJ, Foley KT, Morrow BR, et al. In vitro biomechanics of cervical disc arthroplasty with the Prodisc-C total disc implant. Neurosurg Focus 2004;17(3):E7.

33. Chang UK, Kim DH, Lee MC, et al. Range of motion change after cervical arthroplasty with Prodisc-C and prestige artificial discs compared with anterior cervical discectomy and fusion. J Neurosurg Spine 2007;7(1):40–6.

34. Maldonado C, Paz R, Martin C. Adjacent-level degeneration after cervical disc arthroplasty versus fusion. Eur Spine J 2011;20(Suppl 3):403–7.

35. Nunley P, Jawahar A, Kerr EJ 3rd, et al. Factors affecting the incidence of symptomatic adjacent level disease in cervical spine after total disc arthroplasty: 2–4 years follow-up of 3 prospective randomized trials. Spine (Phila Pa 1976) 2011. [Epub ahead of print].

36. Jawahar A, Cavanaugh D, Kerr E, et al. Total disc arthroplasty does not affect the incidence of adjacent segment degeneration in cervical spine: results of 93 patients in three prospective randomized clinical trials. Spine J 2010;10(12):1043–8.

37. Buchowski J, Anderson P, Sekhon L, et al. Cervical disc arthroplasty compared with arthrodesis for the treatment of myelopathy. Surgical technique. J Bone Joint Surg Am 2009;91(Suppl 2):223–32.

38. Shin D, Yi S, Yoon DH, et al. Artificial disc replacement combined with fusion versus two-level fusion in cervical two-level disc disease. Spine (Phila Pa 1976) 2009;34(11):1153–9 [discussion: 1160–1].

39. Lee M, Dumonski M, Phillips F, et al. Disc replacement adjacent to cervical fusion: a biomechanical comparison of hybrid construct vs. two-level fusion. Spine (Phila Pa 1976) 2011. [Epub ahead of print].

40. Fraser J, Härtl R. Anterior approaches to fusion of the cervical spine: a metaanalysis of fusion rates. J Neurosurg Spine 2007;6(4):298–303.

41. Park Y, Maeda T, Cho W, et al. Comparison of anterior cervical fusion after two-level discectomy or single-level corpectomy: sagittal alignment, cervical lordosis, graft collapse, and adjacent-level ossification. Spine J 2010;10(3):193–9.

42. Wang J, McDonough P, Endow K, et al. A comparison of fusion rates between single-level cervical corpectomy and two-level discectomy and fusion. J Spinal Disord 2001;14(3):222–5.

43. Guo Q, Bi X, Ni B, et al. Outcomes of three anterior decompression and fusion techniques in the treatment of three-level cervical spondylosis. Eur Spine J 2011;20(9):1539–44.

44. Sonntag V, Han P, Vishteh A. Anterior cervical discectomy. Neurosurgery 2001;49(4):909–12.

45. Samartzis D, Shen F, Goldberg E, et al. Is autograft the gold standard in achieving radiographic fusion in one-level anterior cervical discectomy and fusion with rigid anterior plate fixation? Spine (Phila Pa 1976) 2005;30(15):1756–61.

46. Wang J, McDonough P, Endow K, et al. The effect of cervical plating on single-level anterior cervical discectomy and fusion. J Spinal Disord 1999;12(6):467–71.

47. Samartzis D, Shen F, Matthews D, et al. Comparison of allograft to autograft in multilevel anterior cervical discectomy and fusion with rigid plate fixation. Spine J 2003;3(6):451–9.

48. Sevki K, Mehmet T, Ufuk T, et al. Results of surgical treatment for degenerative cervical myelopathy: anterior cervical corpectomy and stabilization. Spine (Phila Pa 1976) 2004;29(22):2493–500.

49. Hwang S, Lee K, Su Y, et al. Anterior corpectomy with iliac bone fusion or discectomy with interbody titanium cage fusion for multilevel cervical degenerated disc disease. J Spinal Disord Tech 2007;20(8):565–70.

50. Lu J, Wu X, Li Y, et al. Surgical results of anterior corpectomy in the aged patients with cervical myelopathy. Eur Spine J 2008;17(1):129–35.

51. Bilbao G, Duart M, Aurrecoechea J, et al. Surgical results and complications in a series of 71

consecutive cervical spondylotic corpectomies. Acta Neurochir (Wien) 2010;152(7):1155–63.

52. Mayr M, Subach B, Comey C, et al. Cervical spinal stenosis: outcome after anterior corpectomy, allograft reconstruction, and instrumentation. J Neurosurg 2002;96(Suppl 1):10–6.

53. Cheng N, Lau P, Sun L, et al. Fusion rate of anterior cervical plating after corpectomy. J Orthop Surg (Hong Kong) 2005;13(3):223–7.

54. Acosta FJ, Aryan H, Chou D, et al. Long-term biomechanical stability and clinical improvement after extended multilevel corpectomy and circumferential reconstruction of the cervical spine using titanium mesh cages. J Spinal Disord Tech 2008; 21(3):165–74.

55. Sasso R, Ruggiero RJ, Reilly T, et al. Early reconstruction failures after multilevel cervical corpectomy. Spine 2003;28(2):140–2.

56. Vaccaro A, Falatyn S, Scuderi G, et al. Early failure of long segment anterior cervical plate fixation. J Spinal Disord 1998;11(5):410–5.

57. Hussain M, Nassr A, Natarajan R, et al. Biomechanical effects of anterior, posterior, and combined anterior-posterior instrumentation techniques on the stability of a multilevel cervical corpectomy construct: a finite element model analysis. Spine J 2011;11(4):324–30.

58. Koller H, Schmidt R, Mayer M, et al. The stabilizing potential of anterior, posterior and combined techniques for the reconstruction of a 2-level cervical corpectomy model: biomechanical study and first results of ATPS prototyping. Eur Spine J 2010; 19(12):2137–48.

59. Epstein N. Anterior approaches to cervical spondylosis and ossification of the posterior longitudinal ligament: review of operative technique and assessment of 65 multilevel circumferential procedures. Surg Neurol 2001;55(6):313–24.

60. Emery S, Bolesta M, Banks M, et al. Robinson anterior cervical fusion comparison of the standard and modified techniques. Spine (Phila Pa 1976) 1994; 19(6):660–3.

61. Brodke D, Gollogly S, Alexander Mohr R, et al. Dynamic cervical plates: biomechanical evaluation of load sharing and stiffness. Spine 2001;26:1324–9.

62. Brodke D, Klimo PJ, Bachus K, et al. Anterior cervical fixation: analysis of load-sharing and stability with use of static and dynamic plates. J Bone Joint Surg Am 2006;88:1566–73.

63. Fogel G, Li Z, Liu W, et al. In vitro evaluation of stiffness and load sharing in a two-level corpectomy: comparison of static and dynamic cervical plates. Spine J 2010;10(5):417–21.

64. Nunley P, Jawahar A, Kerr E, et al. Choice of plate may affect outcomes for single versus multilevel ACDF: results of a prospective randomized single-blind trial. Spine J 2009;9(2):121–7.

65. Koller H, Reynolds J, Zenner J, et al. Mid- to long-term outcome of instrumented anterior cervical fusion for subaxial injuries. Eur Spine J 2009; 18(5):630–53.

66. Park JB, Cho YS, Riew KD. Development of adjacent-level ossification in patients with an anterior cervical plate. J Bone Joint Surg Am 2005;87: 558–63.

67. DuBois CM, Bolt PM, Todd AG, et al. Static versus dynamic plating for multilevel anterior cervical discectomy and fusion. Spine J 2007;7:188–93.

68. Yonenobu K, Hosono N, Iwasaki M, et al. Neurologic complications of surgery for cervical compression myelopathy. Spine (Phila Pa 1976) 1991;16(11):1277–82.

69. Kadoya S, Nakamura T, Kwak R, et al. Anterior osteophytectomy for cervical spondylotic myelopathy in developmentally narrow canal. J Neurosurg 1985;63(6):845–50.

70. Yonenobu K, Okada K, Fuji T, et al. Causes of neurologic deterioration following surgical treatment of cervical myelopathy. Spine 1986;11(8): 818–23.

71. Wang X, Chen Y, Chen D, et al. Removal of posterior longitudinal ligament in anterior decompression for cervical spondylotic myelopathy. J Spinal Disord Tech 2009;22(6):404–7.

72. Connolly E, Seymour R, Adams J. Clinical evaluation of anterior cervical fusion for degenerative cervical disc disease. J Neurosurg 1965;23(4): 431–7.

73. Stevens J, Clifton A, Whitear P. Appearances of posterior osteophytes after sound anterior interbody fusion in the cervical spine: a high-definition computed myelographic study. Neuroradiology 1993;35(3):227–8.

74. Beutler W, Sweeney C, Connolly P. Recurrent laryngeal nerve injury with anterior cervical spine surgery risk with laterality of surgical approach. Spine (Phila Pa 1976) 2001;26(12):1337–42.

75. Kilburg C, Sullivan H, Mathiason M. Effect of approach side during anterior cervical discectomy and fusion on the incidence of recurrent laryngeal nerve injury. J Neurosurg Spine 2006;4(4):273–7.

76. Rihn J, Kane J, Albert T, et al. What is the incidence and severity of dysphagia after anterior cervical surgery? Clin Orthop Relat Res 2011; 469(3):658–65.

77. Riley LH 3rd, Skolasky R, Albert T, et al. Dysphagia after anterior cervical decompression and fusion: prevalence and risk factors from a longitudinal cohort study. Spine (Phila Pa 1976) 2005;30(22): 2564–9.

78. Lee M, Bazaz R, Furey C, et al. Influence of anterior cervical plate design on dysphagia: a 2-year prospective longitudinal follow-up study. J Spinal Disord Tech 2005;18(5):406–9.

79. Shinomiya K, Kurosa Y, Fuchioka M, et al. Clinical study of dissociated motor weakness following anterior cervical decompression surgery. Spine (Phila Pa 1976) 1989;14:1211–4.

80. Tsuzuki N, Tanaka H, Abe R, et al. Cervical radiculopathy occurring after the posterior decompression of the cervical spinal cord. Rinsho Seikei Geka 1991;26:525–34 [in Japanese].

81. Tsuzuki N, Abe R, Saiki K, et al. Extradural tethering effect as one mechanism of radiculopathy complicating posterior decompression of the cervical spinal cord. Spine 1996;21:203–11.

82. Ikenaga M, Shikata J, Tanaka C. Radiculopathy of C-5 after anterior decompression for cervical myelopathy. J Neurosurg Spine 2005;3(3):210–7.

83. Wada E, Suzuki S, Kanazawa A, et al. Subtotal corpectomy versus laminoplasty for multilevel cervical spondylotic myelopathy: a long-term follow- up study over 10 years. Spine 2001;26:1443–8.

84. Hashimoto M, Mochizuki M, Aiba A, et al. C5 palsy following anterior decompression and spinal fusion for cervical degenerative diseases. Eur Spine J 2010;19(10):1702–10.

85. Rueth N, Shaw D, Groth S, et al. Management of cervical esophageal injury after spinal surgery. Ann Thorac Surg 2010;90(4):1128–33.

86. Patel N, Wolcott W, Johnson J, et al. Esophageal injury associated with anterior cervical spine surgery. Surg Neurol 2008;69(1):20–4 [discussion: 24].

87. Chagas H, Domingues F, Aversa A, et al. Cervical spondylotic myelopathy: 10 years of prospective outcome analysis of anterior decompression and fusion. Surg Neurol 2005;64(Suppl 1):S1:30–5 [discussion: S1:35–6].

88. Rajshekhar V, Kumar G. Functional outcome after central corpectomy in poor-grade patients with cervical spondylotic myelopathy or ossified posterior longitudinal ligament. Neurosurgery 2005;56: 1279–84.

89. Chibbaro S, Benvenuti L, Carnesecchi S, et al. Anterior cervical corpectomy for cervical spondylotic myelopathy: experience and surgical results in a series of 70 consecutive patients. J Clin Neurosci 2006;13:233–8.

90. Gok B, Sciubba D, McLoughlin G, et al. Surgical treatment of cervical spondylotic myelopathy with anterior compression: a review of 67 cases. J Neurosurg Spine 2008;9(2):152–7.

91. Sorar M, Seçkin H, Hatipoglu C, et al. Cervical compression myelopathy: is fusion the main prognostic indicator? J Neurosurg Spine 2007;6(6): 531–9.

92. Sakai K, Okawa A, Takahashi M, et al. 5-year follow-up evaluation of surgical treatment for cervical myelopathy caused by ossification of the posterior longitudinal ligament: a prospective comparative study of anterior decompression and fusion with floating method versus laminoplasty. Spine (Phila Pa 1976) 2011. [Epub ahead of print].

93. Furlan J, Kalsi-Ryan S, Kailaya-Vasan A, et al. Functional and clinical outcomes following surgical treatment in patients with cervical spondylotic myelopathy: a prospective study of 81 cases. J Neurosurg Spine 2011;14(3):348–55.

94. Nagashima H, Dokai T, Hashiguchi H, et al. Clinical features and surgical outcomes of cervical spondylotic myelopathy in patients aged 80 years or older: a multi-center retrospective study. Eur Spine J 2011;20(2):240–6.

95. Zhang P, Shen Y, Zhang Y, et al. Significance of increased signal intensity on MRI in prognosis after surgical intervention for cervical spondylotic myelopathy. J Clin Neurosci 2011;18(8): 1080–3.

96. Cho Y, Shin J, Kim K, et al. The relevance of intramedullary high signal intensity and gadolinium (GD-DTPA) enhancement to the clinical outcome in cervical compressive myelopathy. Eur Spine J 2011. [Epub ahead of print].

97. Bertalanffy H, Eggert HR. Complications of anterior cervical discectomy without fusion in 450 consecutive patients. Acta Neurochir (Wien) 1989;99(1–2): 41–50.

98. Emery SE, Bohlman HH, Bolesta MJ, et al. Anterior cervical decompression and arthrodesis for the treatment of cervical spondylotic myelopathy: two to seventeen-year follow-up. J Bone Joint Surg Am 1998;80:941–51.

99. Edwards CC II, Karpitskaya Y, Cha C, et al. Accurate identification of adverse outcomes after cervical spine surgery. J Bone Joint Surg Am 2004;86:251–6.

100. Wang JC, Hart RA, Emery SE, et al. Graft migration or displacement after multilevel cervical corpectomy and strut grafting. Spine 2003;28: 1016–22.

Management of Adjacent Segment Disease After Cervical Spinal Fusion

Christopher K. Kepler, MD, MBA[a],*, Alan S. Hilibrand, MD[b]

KEYWORDS

- Adjacent segment disease • Spinal fusion • Management
- Total disk replacement

Anterior cervical decompression and fusion (ACDF) surgery for cervical spondylosis is often considered to be one of the most successful and predictable procedures that spinal surgeons perform, with high success rates reported in the literature[1–4] at short-term or medium-term follow-up. Despite the relative success of this intervention, one potential source of postoperative pain and disability is symptomatic degeneration at adjacent spinal levels or adjacent segment disease (ASD). This phenomenon was first described clinically in the lumbar spine[5] after several biomechanical cadaveric studies suggested that the greater demands placed on intervertebral disks adjacent to fused vertebrae may lead to accelerated disk degeneration. Subsequently, the same phenomenon was described in the cervical spine after ACDF.[6] In addition to the biomechanical explanation, other potential causes of ASD include injury to musculotendinous, disk, or bony structures during index surgery and natural progression of spondylosis leading to new symptom onset.

ASD has been defined[6] as the "development of new radiculopathy or myelopathy referable to a motion segment adjacent to the site of a previous anterior arthrodesis of the cervical spine." This definition does not require that new symptoms are treated surgically. Symptoms treated surgically, those treated with procedures such as epidural injections, and symptoms treated nonsurgically may all qualify so long as the symptoms are related to an adjacent motion segment based on clinical and radiographic evaluation. In contrast, the similar but distinct concept of adjacent segment degeneration involves the development of new radiographic evidence of spondylosis at a motion segment adjacent to a prior fusion with or without associated symptoms. Despite the clear definition between these 2 terms, they are often used interchangeably in the literature. The reoperation rate cannot typically be used as a proxy for ASD; reoperation may address incomplete decompression at the index level, new pathology at the index level that was not present at index surgery, or new pathology at adjacent or noncontiguous levels, each of which has a distinct pathoanatomy and etiology.

Because of the relative frequency with which ACDF is performed, the consequences of ASD may affect many patients. In recent years, more than 200,000 primary ACDF procedures have been performed annually in the United States.[7] If data from studies with the longest available follow-up after ACDF are correct and the rate of secondary surgery for ASD at 10 years is more than 15%,[6,8,9] a rough calculation suggests that more than 30,000 patients may require surgery for ASD on an annual basis, an estimate that could underestimate the need for reoperation if the rate of ACDF continues to increase as the US population ages.

[a] Department of Orthopaedic Surgery, Thomas Jefferson University & Rothman Institute, 1015 Walnut Street, Room 801, Philadelphia, PA 19107, USA
[b] Department of Orthopaedic Surgery, Thomas Jefferson University & Rothman Institute, 925 Chesnut Street, 5th Floor, Philadelphia, PA 19107, USA
* Corresponding author.
E-mail address: chris.kepler@gmail.com

Orthop Clin N Am 43 (2012) 53–62
doi:10.1016/j.ocl.2011.08.003
0030-5898/12/$ – see front matter © 2012 Elsevier Inc. All rights reserved

Because of the potentially large number of patients affected, ASD presents a significant challenge for spine surgeons to develop techniques that minimize its development. When ASD does occur and symptoms cannot be managed through conservative treatment options, revision operations are frequently encumbered by postsurgical scarring and previous instrumentation. This article characterizes the incidence of ASD after both fusion and motion-preserving surgery, discusses potential preventative strategies that can be used at the time of index surgery, reviews the effectiveness of various conservative therapy options, and discusses surgical considerations for treatment of ASD to select a surgical option and optimize results when conservative therapy is ineffective.

CLINICAL EVIDENCE OF ASD
ASD After ACDF

When studying ASD, clinical research must have a sufficient duration of follow-up to capture the time period during which ASD develops. Although studies with short-term follow-up have occasionally described substantial rates of ASD,[10] most series with short-term follow-up describe high success rates after ACDF[1–4] and 1 or 2 years of surveillance is typically not sufficient to document ASD. With the passage of time, however, adjacent-level degeneration, which is often clinically silent initially,[11] leads to associated symptoms; the need for reoperation at adjacent levels is commonly described in articles with longer follow-up. Thus, long-term studies after ACDF provide the most accurate evaluation of the incidence of ASD. Gore and Sepic[8] described a series of 50 patients who were followed up for an average of 21 years after uninstrumented ACDF. Sixteen of the 50 patients had significant recurrent symptoms and 8 patients required surgery for degeneration at an adjacent level. The 8 patients who had recurrent symptoms but did not require surgery are not described in detail, so it is unclear whether these patients had same-level or different-level spine pathology. The rate of ASD thus lies between 16% and 32%. Hilibrand and colleagues[6] specifically set out to characterize ASD in a series of 374 patients who underwent ACDF. This investigation clearly describes ASD treated both operatively and nonoperatively; in total, ASD developed after 14.2% of the ACDF procedures included in the study, which included 7.2% of patients who underwent secondary surgery. Hilibrand and colleagues reported an annual incidence of 2.9% and estimated the prevalence of ASD at 10 years to be approximately 25%. Ishihara and colleagues[12] performed a study of 112 patients with an average

follow-up of more than 9 years, documenting ASD in 19 patients (17%), including 7 (6.3%) who underwent a second surgery at an adjacent level. Yue and colleagues[9] similarly described the need for reoperation due to ASD in 12/71 (17%) patients treated with ACDF at a follow-up of 7.2 years. Assuming an annualized rate of between 2% and 3%, long-term studies are necessary to accurately study ASD because most studies with short follow-up will not demonstrate stable rates of ASD.

Degeneration in the Native and Unfused Cervical Spine

The intervertebral disk begins to degenerate before any other part of the musculoskeletal system[13] and reliably distinguishing ASD from the natural history of progressive spinal degeneration over time is difficult, especially in an individual with spondylosis severe enough to warrant the index surgery. Some insight into the question of whether ASD occurs after spinal fusion above and beyond the rate of degeneration expected without the influence of spinal fusion can be gained from the study of the natural history of patients treated either without surgery or without fusion. Although these studies could potentially provide a rough approximation of the rate of developing symptomatic cervical spondylosis unrelated to fusion, results have been variable. Gore[14] described a series of 159 individuals without any symptoms referable to the cervical spine who were followed up longitudinally for 10 years with radiographs and clinical history. During this time period, 15% of the participants developed symptoms related to their cervical spine. In addition, Gore identified degenerative changes at C6-C7 on initial examination as a factor that increased the risk of subsequent development of symptomatic cervical spondylosis by more than 4-fold, suggesting C6-C7 should be evaluated carefully before surgery in patients set to undergo single-level ACDF at C5-C6 or C7-T1. Acikbas and colleagues[15] performed a retrospective study of 32 patients treated with anterior cervical diskectomy without attempted fusion for myelopathy and/or radiculopathy with an average postoperative follow-up of 4.8 years. At final follow-up, 8 patients (25%) had developed symptoms attributed to adjacent-level disease. The rate of ASD was nearly identical for a cohort included in the same study treated via posterior cervical fusion (23%), suggesting that ASD was not exclusively related to the anterior approach or associated injury to anterior musculature or osteoligamentous structures. Clarke and colleagues[16] presented a series of patients who developed ASD after posterior spinal foraminotomy. At a follow-up of 7.1 years, 15 patients (4.9% of the cohort of 303 patients) were treated for ASD and the investigators estimated a 10-year follow-up rate of 6.7%. Although the investigators suggested that this rate approached the rate of development of symptoms related to cervical spondylosis at a native motion segment, this study only identified ASD for patients who followed up at the institution where the study was performed and did not contact patients to inquire about treatment elsewhere, likely underestimating the ASD rate.

Factors Influencing ASD After ACDF

Multiple studies have attempted to identify factors that are related to the development of ASD after ACDF. Lower cervical levels have been found to have higher rates of ASD when not included in the index fusion. Hilibrand and colleagues[6] described significantly higher rates of ASD at C5-C6 and C6-C7, the same motion segments that have the highest rates of degeneration in the native spine,[17] and identified increased motion in levels that later degenerated. These findings linking pathologic instability and degeneration have been both supported[10] and refuted[18] by subsequent studies. Hilibrand and colleagues suggested using careful presurgical evaluation of these segments to consider extension of fusion when planning a single-level fusion with preexisting degeneration at C5-C6 or C6-C7 in order to prevent ASD. In a retrospective review comparing patients who had undergone ACDF with asymptomatic volunteers, Matsumoto and colleagues[19] similarly found that patients had a higher likelihood of degenerative changes at adjacent levels 10 years after lower cervical ACDF (C5-C6 or below) compared with those who had undergone ACDF at more cranial levels. Matsumoto and colleagues found, however, that preexisting degenerative changes were not predictive of degeneration at final follow-up, a finding supported by other researchers,[18,20] although it must be noted that this is only a radiographic study. There seems to be little consensus about the importance of preexisting degeneration and increased motion in the progression of radiographic degeneration, although relative strengths of the Hilibrand study[6] are substantially longer follow-up and evaluation of clinical symptoms rather than just degenerative changes on imaging.

ASD After Total Disk Replacement

At present, there is insufficient clinical data time to thoroughly evaluate the theoretic advantages of motion preservation technology in preventing ASD. Clinical data from ACDF studies have more

clearly implicated the natural history of specific motion segments rather than the effect of pathologic motion, but it remains to be seen whether studies on motion-preserving implants will draw similar conclusions. Regardless, the prevention of ASD was one of the primary rationales for the development of motion-preserving technologies. Motion-preserving surgical options, such as total disk replacement (TDR), have been studied to determine if the theoretic advantages for adjacent motion segments can be realized in clinical practice. Several short-term and medium-term follow-up studies have been published from the Investigational Device Exemption (IDE) trials associated with the US Food and Drug Administration approval process for TDR. Because these trials were designed to compare TDR with ACDF, the study cohorts provide an opportunity to compare TDR with ACDF in terms of ASD rate and factors associated with the development of ASD.

The IDE studies enrolled patients with single-level radiculopathy or myelopathy in need of single-level decompression; patients were randomized to either ACDF or TDR. Early reports from these investigations seemed to favor TDR. Two-year data from Mummaneni and colleagues[21] comparing patients treated with ACDF with those treated using the Prestige TDR reported significantly higher rates of surgical intervention for ASD (3.4% vs 1.1%, $P = .049$). Only surgical intervention for ASD was reported; more rigorous methods of identifying ASD that did not require surgery were not used. The investigators attributed the decreased ASD rate to differential maintenance of physiologic motion after ACDF (allowing excessive supraphysiologic motion) and TDR (motion similar to preoperative range). More recent publications have shown less difference between ACDF and TDR in terms of ASD. In 2010, Burkus and colleagues[22] presented a 5-year follow-up from the same Prestige cohort previously described 2 years after index surgery by Mummaneni and colleagues.[21] At the most recent follow-up, the incidence of ASD requiring reoperation was similar between the ACDF and TDR groups, although this study had less power to detect a difference because of the smaller group size (271 total patients in this study vs 421 in the previous report). Jawahar and colleagues[23] used a more rigorous definition of ASD in their study of 93 patients enrolled in IDE TDA trials at an average follow-up of just over 3 years and found no significant difference in the rate of ASD between ACDF (15%) and TDR (18%). Nunley and colleagues[24] also found no difference between patients with ACDF (14%) and those with TDR (17%) who were actively treated for ASD at an average follow-up of 42 months. These last 2 studies likely contain many of the same patients based on the description of the study populations and author list but Nunley and colleagues[24] do include an additional 77 patients and a 3-month longer follow-up. A 3-year follow-up after TDR was recently presented and showed a statistically significant decrease in ASD in the TDR group compared with the ACDF control group.[25] The best available evidence currently does not present a clear picture to compare the rate of ASD between ACDF and cervical TDR; a longer-term follow-up is needed.

Jawahar and colleagues[23] and Nunley and colleagues[24] identified the presence of lumbar spondylosis as a patient-related factor associated with ASD. These studies used multiple regression methodologies for identification of factors influencing the rate of ASD, so these findings are independent of procedure; lumbar degeneration influences ASD regardless of whether a patient undergoes ACDF or TDR. This finding is consistent with contemporary evidence about factors affecting susceptibility to disk degeneration suspected to be largely dominated by genetics, which may be responsible for more than 75% of individual susceptibility to symptomatic degeneration.[26,27] Nunley and colleagues[24] also identified osteopenia as a procedure-independent factor contributing to susceptibility to ASD.

PRINCIPLES OF MANAGEMENT OF ASD
Preoperative Prevention Strategies

Spine surgeons evaluating patients with cervical radiculopathy or myelopathy for ACDF should pay careful attention to the history and physical examination to accurately characterize the levels involved. Updated imaging studies are similarly important to accurately identify symptom-generating motion segments, particularly for the lower cervical levels, which have greater native motion arcs,[28] and have been shown to be more susceptible to degeneration in the native spine as described earlier. In this sense, the spinal surgeon must accurately identify all levels causing bothersome symptoms without being overly aggressive and operating on an asymptomatic degenerative disk.

The importance of including adjacent degenerative levels in the index procedure has been demonstrated by Hilibrand and colleagues[6] who described a higher rate of ASD in patients who underwent single-level surgery. Although this finding initially seems contrary to explanations implicating lever arm length and associated pathologic adjacent-level disk stresses in the pathogenesis of ASD, this phenomenon is more likely related to undertreating patients who have multilevel disease using a single-level operation. Confirmatory evidence of this effect was presented by Komura and colleagues,[29] who studied patients treated with long or short ACDF constructs that did or did not include the C5 to C7 motion segments, respectively. This study demonstrated an increased rate of ASD in the patients treated with longer fusions, indicating that the specific levels included in the index procedure are important in ASD; the lever arm may be of secondary importance to preexisting degeneration or susceptibility to degeneration in the development of ASD.

Intraoperative Prevention Strategies

Surgeons should attempt to limit the iatrogenic zone of soft-tissue injury during ACDF as much as possible to maintain the supporting role that musculoligamentous structures play in regulating normal intervertebral disk mobility. The longus colli is a longitudinal structure with fibers that span between multiple spinal levels and may impart substantial dynamic stability to the intervertebral disk.[30,31] Dissection along the anterior vertebral border should be performed using a minimally disruptive technique and should focus on elevating, not transecting, the muscle fibers to reduce the effect on adjacent levels. When anterior plating is performed as an adjunct to ACDF, the use of a shorter plate facilitates minimal muscle dissection. The surgeon must also be particularly careful not to inadvertently injure the adjacent disk itself in any way during dissection or application of the plate. The disk has a poor capacity for regeneration and any significant injury will likely result in accelerated degeneration. Recently, this susceptibility to injury was demonstrated by an investigation in which even needle annulotomy associated with incorrect intraoperative level localization before diskectomy resulted in a 3-fold increase in degeneration.[32]

Impingement of an anterior plate on an adjacent level may cause adjacent-level ossification disease (ALOD) as initially described by Park and colleagues.[33] ALOD has been proposed to result from irritation and disruption of soft-tissue structures, such as the anterior longitudinal ligament or the anterior fibers of the annulus fibrosus.[33,34] The severity of ALOD can range from minor involvement with focal ossification to bridging bone, which can eliminate adjacent-level motion in severe cases. Maintaining a vertical distance between the edge of the plate and the vertebral end plate of at least 5 mm has been demonstrated empirically to substantially reduce the incidence of ALOD.[35] The avoidance of unnecessary disruption of the musculoligamentous structures along the anterior vertebral border, the reduced risk of direct injury to the disk during dissection, and the ability to maintain a safe margin between the plate edge and adjacent vertebrae all suggest that ACDF may be optimized by placement of a short plate with screws angled away from the plate, if possible, to maximize screw purchase and minimize iatrogenic soft-tissue injury.

Conservative Management Options

Because many studies focus discussion of ASD on patients treated surgically, it is often difficult to discern the success of conservative treatment. Hilibrand and colleagues[6] followed up 46 patients for 2 or more years after the development of ASD; all patients with ASD were initially treated conservatively. Of these, 13 patients (28%) were successfully managed with conservative treatment (soft cervical collar, physiotherapy, and antiinflammatory medications) and achieved good or excellent outcomes. Six patients (13%) either refused surgery or were not offered revision and all had fair outcomes. The remaining patients (59%) failed conservative treatment and required ACDF of the adjacent level. In a smaller series, Elsawaf and colleagues[10] were able to successfully treat 4 of the 5 patients who developed ASD after ACDF using conservative methods, although no information is provided about their conservative treatment protocol and the average follow-up averaged only 28 months. Similarly, Acikbas and colleagues[15] found that all 19 patients who developed ASD after cervical fusion responded to an "aggressive regimen of conservative therapy" and avoided surgery. Closer investigation, however, demonstrates that 18 of these 19 patients developed ASD at 5 years or more after the index surgery. Given the average follow-up for the study was only 4.8 years, the duration of successful conservative treatment must have been short; longer follow-up may spoil these promising results after conservative treatment. More evidence is needed to determine if ASD can be reliably treated nonsurgically or if the previous history of spondylosis is associated with an accelerated clinical course for the degenerative adjacent level that frequently results in reoperation. As when treating the initial onset of radiculopathy or neck pain in the native cervical spine, conservative treatment best practice is ill-defined. A wide variety of protocols using physical therapy, limited immobilization, traction, antiinflammatory medications, and injections have been used in combination or individually with little literature to support any one treatment strategy.

OPERATING FOR ASD
Selecting an Approach

In those patients who have failed conservative treatment, the spine surgeon must select a surgical approach to address the symptomatic degenerative motion segment. As with primary procedures, decompression and/or fusion can be performed using anterior, posterior, or anterior/posterior approaches.

After a successful index surgery with radiographic evidence of fusion, the anterior approach is most often selected for treatment of ASD for either central canal or lateral recess stenosis at 1 or 2 adjacent levels. Although there is mounting evidence regarding the efficacy of TDR for ASD, ACDF is more familiar to most surgeons and has a larger body of supporting literature.

In a retrospective review of 38 patients treated for ASD after ACDF, Hilibrand and colleagues[36] described 24 patients treated with a second ACDF procedure at 1, 2, or 3 levels and 14 patients treated with corpectomy for 2-, 3-, or 4-level ASD. At a follow-up of 68 months, the investigators found that 32 of the 38 patients (84%) had self-described excellent or good outcomes. Patients had a better outcome overall when treated with corpectomy compared with ACDF and the study demonstrated a trend toward improved outcome in patients who went on to successful fusion of their adjacent motion segment. Gause and colleagues[37] published results for 56 patients treated with either ACDF or corpectomy and fusion for ASD after ACDF. Although this study did not use patient-centered outcome measures, 84% of patients achieved fusion after 1-level ACDF for ASD, whereas 2-level secondary procedures resulted in a fusion rate of 80%. In the 49 patients treated with ACDF, 81% achieved fusion compared with 100% of the 7 patients treated with corpectomy, echoing the results described by Hilibrand and colleagues.[36] Of the 9 patients who went on to nonunion, 3 ultimately underwent a third procedure to place supplemental posterior fixation; 1 patient still had significant symptoms associated with nonunion at final follow-up. A small series published by Arnold and colleagues[38] described 7 patients treated for ASD with placement of a threaded cylindrical cage without plating. All patients achieved good or excellent results, had a greater than 4-point improvement on the visual analog scale (VAS) for neck and arm pain, a 12.3-point improvement in the Neck Disability Index, and achieved fusion at a follow-up of 24 months. The investigators described potential advantages of the surgical approach used in their series, including minimal dissection along the anterior vertebrae borders; the use of a cylindrical cage and not placing an anterior plate minimized the exposure and the need for dissection in the scarred surgical bed.

Although ACDF has a longer track record, TDR has also been used to treat patients with ASD at either 1 or 2 levels although there is less available literature to provide guidance. Sekhon and colleagues[39] included 9 patients who had undergone 1- or 2-level TDR for ASD after ACDF in a series of 15 patients treated with TDR after previous surgery (the remaining 6 patients had previous posterior cervical foraminotomy). Although results are not broken down by index procedure type, overall VAS improved by 6.4 and Oswestry Disability Index improved by 9.5 points at an average follow-up of 19 months. One patient had asymptomatic excessive motion after TDR for ASD but did not require intervention. The segmental alignment at treated motion segments lost 4° of lordosis on average after TDR. Phillips and colleagues[40] described 26 patients treated with single-level disk replacement for ASD after ACDF and compared this cohort with a group of patients undergoing TDR as a primary surgery. At a follow-up of 1 year, Neck Disability Index scores, VAS pain scores, and revision rates were similar, suggesting that the use of TDR for ASD is as efficacious as primary TDR in the short term. Shin and colleagues[41] provide indirect support for the use of TDR after ACDF in their study of 40 patients treated for 2-level spondylosis with radiculopathy with either 2-level ACDF or ACDF-TDR hybrid surgery. Although both levels were treated simultaneously, this study may still provide insight into the comparative postoperative outcome and biomechanical parameters associated with 2-level ACDF versus ACDF-TDR. Neck Disability Index scores improved significantly more in the hybrid group, as did neck pain, compared with the 2-level ACDF group. On addition, the inferior adjacent level demonstrated hypermobility in the ACDF group versus hypomobility in the hybrid group, which may slow the development of ASD, although this effect has only been supported by biomechanical studies,[42] not clinically. Although this study describes simultaneous 2-level surgery instead of staged surgery due to interval development of ASD, it does suggest potential clinical and biomechanical advantages of a fusion-TDR construct.

Procedures using the posterior approach should be considered when decompression and fusion are required at more than 2 levels as a result of ASD in patients with intact cervical lordosis or in patients with minimal adjacent-level spondylosis when foraminotomy or laminoplasty may be a treatment option. Patients who are congenitally stenotic and present with multilevel compression may be treated with either laminoplasty or laminectomy and fusion. Several investigators have described the outcomes after laminoplasty to treat ASD. Baba and colleagues[43] published an early series describing 18 patients treated with laminoplasty for ASD after ACDF and followed up for an average of 2.8 years. The investigators used the Japanese Orthopaedic Association assessment scoring system to evaluate the patients postoperatively and demonstrated 10 good/excellent results (56%), with a greater proportion of good/excellent results in men and in patients with a longer symptom-free period before presentation with ASD. Matsumoto and colleagues[44] also found improvement after open-door laminoplasty for myelopathic ASD but a matched control population of patients undergoing primary surgery for myelopathy demonstrated greater gains in the Japanese Orthopaedic Association scores. Based on these results, the investigators suggested that patients with ASD may have less potential for improvement because of chronic compression at the affected levels and recommended early intervention when patients present with symptoms of ASD.

Anteroposterior combined approaches for decompression and fusion to treat ASD may be considered for patients presenting with multilevel disease and associated kyphosis to improve the likelihood of fusion after ACDF in patients with significant risk factors for nonunion (eg, smokers) or after demonstrated biological deficiency based on nonunion at the index level, suggesting the patient may benefit from circumferential fusion.

Technical Considerations for Repeat Anterior Surgery

As with all revision anterior cervical surgery, preoperative considerations must include the side of approach to be used. Patients presenting with a single-level ASD can often undergo ACDF through the incision from the index procedure. If the number of levels to be treated or the position of the original incision will preclude the use of the previous incision, then the contralateral side can be used. Before surgery, however, the patient must undergo evaluation of their vocal cords by an otolaryngologist to ensure that their vocal cords are still functional on the side of the original approach. If the index surgery injured the recurrent laryngeal nerve, then surgery should be performed on the same side as the index surgery to avoid aphonia and respiratory dysfunction, which can result from bilateral recurrent laryngeal nerve injury.

The presence of a successful index-level fusion presents theoretic challenges for the adjacent-level surgery. Achieving fusion relies on relative immobility during the early postoperative period and some biomechanical evidence[42,45] suggests that motion segments adjacent to prior fusion have supraphysiologic motion; for this reason, the authors recommend maximizing stiffness through the use of anterior plating when performing ACDF to treat ASD. Increased adjacent-level motion may also increase strain on a TDR placed at an adjacent level. Although such an effect has been suggested based on biomechanical findings,[42] this has not yet been studied clinically in a systematic manner to establish if the use of TDR can prevent ASD or normalize cervical motion. Sekhon and colleagues[39] described 1 patient who demonstrated asymptomatic excessive prosthetic translation after treatment of ASD with TDR, but whether the adjacent fusion contributed to this event is unknown. Further study is needed to identify the optimal strategy for treatment of ASD after ACDF.

SUMMARY

A growing body of literature has improved understanding of ASD after cervical fusion. Although ASD is clearly defined as symptoms of radiculopathy or myelopathy secondary to spondylosis at a motion segment next to a previous fusion, the literature contains many references to ASD based entirely on radiographic signs of degeneration. ASD likely occurs after cervical fusion at a rate of approximately 25% at 10 years after surgery based on the best available evidence. Clinical evidence of the rate of ASD after disk replacement is inconsistent, although studies with longer follow-up report no difference compared with the rate of ASD after ACDF, a finding that would support the argument that ASD is more closely related to a patient's individual susceptibility to cervical spondylosis than to the postsurgical biomechanics of the spine. Nonetheless, careful preoperative consideration to identify all symptomatic levels before index surgery and careful avoidance of iatrogenic soft-tissue injury that could lead to ASD is important to minimize the incidence of ASD. For patients who fail conservative treatment of ASD, both anterior and posterior surgical options may be used although little evidence-based guidance is available at present.

CLINICAL PEARLS

- Spine surgeons should establish patient expectations regarding the possibility of

ASD before index surgery; the best evidence suggests a rate of approximately 25% at 10 years after surgery.
- Careful preoperative clinical and radiographic evaluation is necessary before surgery to make sure that all symptomatic levels are included in the index procedure, particularly in the lower cervical spine where ASD is more common.
- At the time of index surgery, care to avoid unnecessary soft-tissue injury and to protect adjacent disks not involved in the surgery minimize the risk of iatrogenic ASD.
- Anterior plates should be placed more than 5 mm from the vertebral end plates to avoid impinging on unfused, adjacent motion segments.
- There is little evidence to guide a spinal surgeon in treating ASD with ACDF versus TDR but, when performing ACDF, the authors recommend the use of anterior plating to counteract the tendency toward greater motion at motion segments adjacent to a fusion to maximize the likelihood of successful fusion.

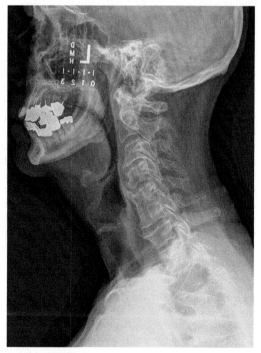

Fig. 1. Preoperative lateral radiograph after C5-C6 diskectomy demonstrating fusion of C5-C6. C4-C5 was also demonstrated to have fused spontaneously on a computed tomography scan (not shown).

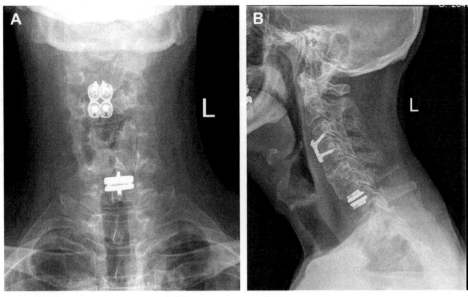

Fig. 2. Postoperative anteroposterior (*A*) and lateral (*B*) radiographs demonstrating TDR at C6-C7 to preserve motion at that level and anterior cervical discectomy and fusion at C3-C4.

CASE HISTORY

The patient is a 51-year-old man who presented 11 years after undergoing C5-C6 anterior cervical diskectomy without attempted fusion for bilateral radiculopathy at another institution. The patient had resolution of his symptoms postoperatively and did well for 9 years. On recent presentation, the patient complained of recurrent radicular symptoms in the left arm and denied any history consistent with myelopathy. Radiographs and computed tomography scan demonstrated spontaneous fusion at the previously operated level, C5-C6, as well as at C4-C5 (**Fig. 1**). Magnetic resonance imaging demonstrated herniated nucleus pulposis with spinal cord compression at C6/C7 and a compressive osteophyte-disk complex at C3-C4. Flexion-extension radiographs demonstrated little motion at C3-C4 but preserved motion at C6-C7. The patient underwent TDR at C6-C7 to attempt to preserve motion at that level and a simultaneous anterior cervical diskectomy and fusion at C3-C4 (**Fig. 2**). The C4 to C6 levels were explored intraoperatively and noted to be fused.

REFERENCES

1. Hacker RJ. A randomized prospective study of an anterior cervical interbody fusion device with a minimum of 2 years of follow-up results. J Neurosurg 2000;93(Suppl 2):222–6.
2. Kaiser MG, Haid RW, Jr, Subach BR, et al. Anterior cervical plating enhances arthrodesis after discectomy and fusion with cortical allograft. Neurosurgery 2002; 50(2):229–36 [discussion: 236–8].
3. Samartzis D, Shen FH, Lyon C, et al. Does rigid instrumentation increase the fusion rate in one-level anterior cervical discectomy and fusion? Spine J 2004;4(6):636–43.
4. Samartzis D, Shen FH, Goldberg EJ, et al. Is autograft the gold standard in achieving radiographic fusion in one-level anterior cervical discectomy and fusion with rigid anterior plate fixation? Spine 2005; 30(15):1756–61.
5. Lee CK. Accelerated degeneration of the segment adjacent to a lumbar fusion. Spine (Phila Pa 1976) 1988;13(3):375–7.
6. Hilibrand AS, Carlson GD, Palumbo MA, et al. Radiculopathy and myelopathy at segments adjacent to the site of a previous anterior cervical arthrodesis. J Bone Joint Surg Am 1999;81(4):519–28.
7. Memtsoudis SG, Hughes A, Ma Y, et al. Increased in-hospital complications after primary posterior versus primary anterior cervical fusion. Clin Orthop Relat Res 2011;469(3):649–57.
8. Gore DR, Sepic SB. Anterior discectomy and fusion for painful cervical disc disease. A report of 50 patients with an average follow-up of 21 years. Spine (Phila Pa 1976) 1998;23(19):2047–51.
9. Yue WM, Brodner W, Highland TR. Long-term results after anterior cervical discectomy and fusion with allograft and plating: a 5- to 11-year radiologic and clinical follow-up study. Spine (Phila Pa 1976) 2005;30(19):2138–44.
10. Elsawaf A, Mastronardi L, Roperto R, et al. Effect of cervical dynamics on adjacent segment degeneration

after anterior cervical fusion with cages. Neurosurg Rev 2009;32(2):215–24 [discussion: 224].

11. Iseda T, Goya T, Nakano S, et al. Serial changes in signal intensities of the adjacent discs on T2-weighted sagittal images after surgical treatment of cervical spondylosis: anterior interbody fusion versus expansive laminoplasty. Acta Neurochir (Wien) 2001;143(7):707–10.

12. Ishihara H, Kanamori M, Kawaguchi Y, et al. Adjacent segment disease after anterior cervical interbody fusion. Spine J 2004;4(6):624–8.

13. Buckwalter JA. Aging and degeneration of the human intervertebral disc. Spine (Phila Pa 1976) 1995;20(11):1307–14.

14. Gore DR. Roentgenographic findings in the cervical spine in asymptomatic persons: a ten-year follow-up. Spine (Phila Pa 1976) 2001;26(22):2463–6.

15. Acikbas SC, Ermol C, Akyuz M, et al. Assessment of adjacent segment degeneration in and between patients treated with anterior or posterior cervical simple discectomy. Turk Neurosurg 2010;20(3): 334–40.

16. Clarke MJ, Ecker RD, Krauss WE, et al. Same-segment and adjacent-segment disease following posterior cervical foraminotomy. J Neurosurg Spine 2007;6(1):5–9.

17. Boden SD, McCowin PR, Davis DO, et al. Abnormal magnetic-resonance scans of the cervical spine in asymptomatic subjects. A prospective investigation. J Bone Joint Surg Am 1990;72(8):1178–84.

18. Reitman CA, Hipp JA, Nguyen L, et al. Changes in segmental intervertebral motion adjacent to cervical arthrodesis: a prospective study. Spine (Phila Pa 1976) 2004;29(11):E221–6.

19. Matsumoto M, Okada E, Ichihara D, et al. Anterior cervical decompression and fusion accelerates adjacent segment degeneration: comparison with asymptomatic volunteers in a ten-year magnetic resonance imaging follow-up study. Spine (Phila Pa 1976) 2010;35(1):36–43.

20. Kolstad F, Nygaard OP, Leivseth G. Segmental motion adjacent to anterior cervical arthrodesis: a prospective study. Spine (Phila Pa 1976) 2007; 32(5):512–7.

21. Mummaneni PV, Burkus JK, Haid RW, et al. Clinical and radiographic analysis of cervical disc arthroplasty compared with allograft fusion: a randomized controlled clinical trial. J Neurosurg Spine 2007;6(3): 198–209.

22. Burkus JK, Haid RW, Traynelis VC, et al. Long-term clinical and radiographic outcomes of cervical disc replacement with the Prestige disc: results from a prospective randomized controlled clinical trial. J Neurosurg Spine 2010;13(3):308–18.

23. Jawahar A, Cavanaugh DA, Kerr EJ 3rd, et al. Total disc arthroplasty does not affect the incidence of adjacent segment degeneration in cervical spine:

results of 93 patients in three prospective randomized clinical trials. Spine J 2010;10(12):1043–8.

24. Nunley PD, Jawahar A, Kerr EJ 3rd, et al. Factors affecting the incidence of symptomatic adjacent level disease in cervical spine after total disc arthroplasty: 2-4 years follow-up of 3 prospective randomized trials. Spine (Phila Pa 1976) 2011. [Epub ahead of print].

25. Murrey D, Janssen M, Delamarter R, et al. 5-year results of the prospective, randomized, multicenter FDA Investigational Device Exemption (IDE) ProDisc-C TDR clinical trial [abstract: #1]. Presented at: Cervical Spine Research Society Annual Meeting. Salt Lake City (UT), December 3–5, 2009.

26. Postacchini F, Lami R, Pugliese O. Familial predisposition to discogenic low-back pain. An epidemiologic and immunogenetic study. Spine (Phila Pa 1976) 1988;13(12):1403–6.

27. Bijkerk C, Houwing-Duistermaat JJ, Valkenburg HA, et al. Heritabilities of radiologic osteoarthritis in peripheral joints and of disc degeneration of the spine. Arthritis Rheum 1999;42(8):1729–35.

28. Johnson RM, Crelin ES, White AA 3rd, et al. Some new observations on the functional anatomy of the lower cervical spine. Clin Orthop Relat Res 1975;(111):192–200.

29. Komura S, Miyamoto K, Hosoe H, et al. Lower incidence of adjacent segment degeneration after anterior cervical fusion found with those fusing C5-6 and C6-7 than those leaving C5-6 or C6-7 as an adjacent level. J Spinal Disord Tech 2011. [Epub ahead of print].

30. Goffin J, van Loon J, Van Calenbergh F, et al. Long-term results after anterior cervical fusion and osteosynthetic stabilization for fractures and/or dislocations of the cervical spine. J Spinal Disord 1995;8(6):500–8 [discussion: 499].

31. Kettler A, Hartwig E, Schultheiss M, et al. Mechanically simulated muscle forces strongly stabilize intact and injured upper cervical spine specimens. J Biomech 2002;35(3):339–46.

32. Nassr A, Lee JY, Bashir RS, et al. Does incorrect level needle localization during anterior cervical discectomy and fusion lead to accelerated disc degeneration? Spine (Phila Pa 1976) 2009;34(2):189–92.

33. Park JB, Cho YS, Riew KD. Development of adjacent-level ossification in patients with an anterior cervical plate. J Bone Joint Surg Am 2005; 87(3):558–63.

34. Yang JY, Song HS, Lee M, et al. Adjacent level ossification development after anterior cervical fusion without plate fixation. Spine (Phila Pa 1976) 2009; 34(1):30–3.

35. Park JB, Watthanaaphisit T, Riew KD. Timing of development of adjacent-level ossification after anterior cervical arthrodesis with plates. Spine J 2007;7(6):633–6.

36. Hilibrand AS, Yoo JU, Carlson GD, et al. The success of anterior cervical arthrodesis adjacent to a previous fusion. Spine (Phila Pa 1976) 1997;22(14):1574–9.

37. Gause PR, Davis RA, Smith PN, et al. Success of junctional anterior cervical discectomy and fusion. Spine J 2008;8(5):723–8.

38. Arnold P, Boswell S, McMahon J. Threaded interbody fusion cage for adjacent segment degenerative disease after previous anterior cervical fusion. Surg Neurol 2008;70(4):390–7.

39. Sekhon LH, Sears W, Duggal N. Cervical arthroplasty after previous surgery: results of treating 24 discs in 15 patients. J Neurosurg Spine 2005;3(5): 335–41.

40. Phillips FM, Allen TR, Regan JJ, et al. Cervical disc replacement in patients with and without previous adjacent level fusion surgery: a prospective study. Spine (Phila Pa 1976) 2009;34(6):556–65.

41. Shin DA, Yi S, Yoon do H, et al. Artificial disc replacement combined with fusion versus two-level fusion in cervical two-level disc disease. Spine (Phila Pa 1976) 2009;34(11):1153–9 [discussion: 1160–1].

42. Cunningham BW, Hu N, Zorn CM, et al. Biomechanical comparison of single- and two-level cervical arthroplasty versus arthrodesis: effect on adjacent-level spinal kinematics. Spine J 2010;10(4):341–9.

43. Baba H, Furusawa N, Imura S, et al. Laminoplasty following anterior cervical fusion for spondylotic myeloradiculopathy. Int Orthop 1994;18(1):1–5.

44. Matsumoto M, Nojiri K, Chiba K, et al. Open-door laminoplasty for cervical myelopathy resulting from adjacent-segment disease in patients with previous anterior cervical decompression and fusion. Spine (Phila Pa 1976) 2006;31(12):1332–7.

45. Park DK, Lin EL, Phillips FM. Index and adjacent level kinematics after cervical disc replacement and anterior fusion: in vivo quantitative radiographic analysis. Spine (Phila Pa 1976) 2011; 36(9):721–30.

Esophageal and Vertebral Artery Injuries During Complex Cervical Spine Surgery— Avoidance and Management

Gregory Grabowski, MD[a],*, Chris A. Cornett, MD[b],
James D. Kang, MD[c]

KEYWORDS

• Vertebral artery • Esophagus • Cervical spine

VERTEBRAL ARTERY ANATOMY

The paired vertebral arteries are branches off of the first portion of each subclavian artery. These arteries are generally unequal in size, with the left the larger and dominant of the two.[1] The typical course of the vertebral artery allows for its classic division into 4 segments, V1 though V4. The first segment (V1) starts with the branching of the vertebral artery from the subclavian artery and follows as it travels anterior to the transverse foramen of C7 and into the transverse foramen of C6. The second segment (V2) includes the section of the artery as it passes through the successive vertebral foramina from C6 to C1. V3 comprises the portion from the superior aspect of the arch of the atlas to the foramen magnum; (V4) extends from the foramen magnum to the confluence with the contralateral vertebral artery and together they form the basilar artery (**Fig. 1**).[2]

Various anatomic relationships throughout the course of the vertebral artery are important to the spine surgeon. In the V2 region, the artery normally remains 1.5 mm or more lateral to the uncovertebral joint.[3] Furthermore, the bony architecture within the region of the V2 segment dictates a mildly convergent course of the arteries through this section; the mean interforaminal distance at C6 is approximately 29 mm compared with 26 mm at C3.[4] Similarly, the mean distance from the medial edge of the longus colli to the medial edge of the vertebral artery decreases from 11.5 mm at C6 to 9 mm at C3.[5] Although the transverse foramina of the subaxial spine are ring-shaped, the transverse foramen of C2 is an angulated canal bordered by the pedicle and lateral mass. Its inferior and lateral openings allow the artery to deviate 45° laterally before continuing its ascent to enter the transverse foramen of C1.[6]

The V3 segment becomes important to the spine surgeon mostly during posterior surgery of the atlantoaxial joint. As the artery exits the foramen of C1, it travels posteriorly and medially inside the vertebral artery groove on the superior

The authors have nothing to disclose.
[a] Department of Orthopaedics and Sports Medicine, University of South Carolina School of Medicine, Two Medical Park, Suite 404, Columbia, SC 29203, USA
[b] Department of Orthopaedic Surgery and Rehabilitation, University of Nebraska Medical Center, 981080 University of Nebraska Medical Center, Omaha, NE 68198-1080, USA
[c] Department of Orthopaedic Surgery, University of Pittsburgh, 3471 Fifth Avenue, Pittsburgh, PA 15213, USA
* Corresponding author.
E-mail address: gregory.grabowski78@gmail.com

Orthop Clin N Am 43 (2012) 63–74
doi:10.1016/j.ocl.2011.08.008

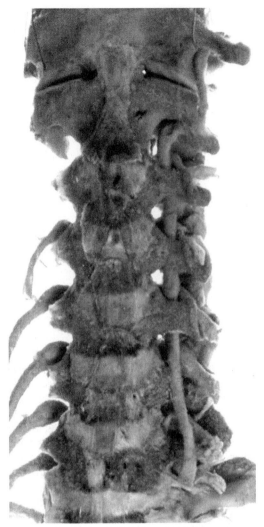

Fig. 1. Gross dissection of the cervical spine demonstrating typical anatomy of the left vertebral artery, including passage anterior to the transverse foramen at C7. The artery subsequently enters the C6 foramen and passes through each successive foraminae to C1.

aspect of the atlas. At a distance ranging from 8 mm to 18 mm from the midline, the artery abruptly changes course, traveling anteriorly and superiorly toward the foramen magnum.[7]

ANOMALOUS VERTEBRAL ARTERY ANATOMY

Although anatomic anomalies within the V2 segment are rare, their presence can be important, particularly in patients undergoing anterior cervical spine surgery. These anomalies can be divided into 3 major categories: intraforaminal, extraforaminal, and arterial.

Intraforaminal anomalies, also known as vertebral artery tortuosity, can be defined as a vertebral artery which is located medial to, or less than 1.5 mm lateral to, the uncovertebral joint.[8] Generally, this refers to the midline migration of the vertebral artery causing erosion into the vertebral body (**Fig. 2**). Several hypotheses have been proposed to explain why such tortuosity occurs. These include degenerative changes and posttraumatic changes as well as less common causes, such as infection, tumor, systemic disease, and prior surgical nonunion.[8–11] Cadaveric studies have shown the incidence of this condition to be 2.7%, with C3 and C4 the most commonly affected levels.[12] More recent MRI-based studies showed a higher incidence, 7.6%, and found that patients with a tortuous vertebral artery tended to be older than patients without this finding (**Fig. 3**).[8]

Extraforaminal anomalies refer to instances where the vertebral artery runs anterior to the transverse foramen at one or multiple levels between C6 and C1. An analysis of CT angiograms showed that the vertebral artery enters through the C6 transverse foramen 94.9% of the time. Anomalous entry sites at C4, C5, and C7, however, occurred at 1.6%, 3.3%, and 0.3%, respectively.[13] In their MRI-based study, Eskander and colleagues[8] found that only 92% of arteries entered at C6 (**Figs. 4** and **5**).

Arterial abnormalities are varied but include such findings as dual-lumen and triple-lumen arteries or the presence of a hypoplastic vertebral artery. Although most of these findings have little surgical implication, vertebral artery hypoplasia affects treatment options and potential neurologic sequelae in the case of an inadvertent injury. Hypoplasia occurs in approximately 10% of the population.[8]

At the atlanto-occipital joint, variations occur with greater regularity. Erosion of the C2 transverse foramen has been reported to have an incidence of 33%, occurring more commonly on the

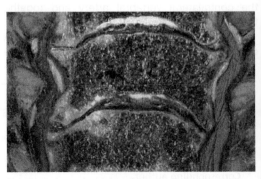

Fig. 2. Gross specimen demonstrating a tortuous vertebral artery with erosion into the lateral vertebral body wall.

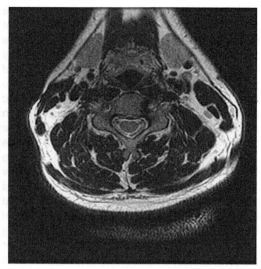

Fig. 3. Axial T2-weighted MRI demonstrating tortuous left vertebral artery with erosion into the vertebral body.

left side.[6] Of these anomalies, 20% are severe enough to preclude the safe placement of C2 instrumentation.[14] Similarly, arcuate foramina of C1 have a reported prevalence of 15.5%, with implications on exposure for C1 lateral mass screw placement.[15]

ANTERIOR SPINE SURGERY

Vertebral artery injury is a rare but profound complication of anterior spinal surgery. Its relative infrequency limits its presence in the literature to case reports or small case series. The largest series of these injuries cite the incidence of injury as approximately 0.3%.[16–19] This midline migration can cause erosion into the vertebral body. An instance of postoperative presentation with a lateral medullary infarct, however, has also been reported in a patient whose only intraoperative finding was "epidural oozing."[18]

In patients with normal vertebral artery anatomy, the artery is most susceptible to injury during anterior procedures in its position anterior to the transverse foramen of C7 or during lateral decompressive maneuvers from C3 to C6. Constant orientation to the anatomic midline is paramount in avoiding injury both during exposure and decompression. The midpoint between the longus colli muscles serves as a reliable intraoperative landmark of the midline, and dissection can safely be performed over the uncovertebral joints. From C3 to C6, the artery is protected by the transverse foramen at the level of the uncovertebral joint, allowing for safe exposure of these structures to their lateral extent; however, care should be taken while exposing the C7 uncovertebral joint given the anterior position of this structure at this level. The presence of an aberrant entry level, however, can place the artery at risk anteriorly at other levels if not recognized preoperatively. At the levels of the vertebral bodies, dissection can safely be carried to the downslope of the vertebrae.[20]

During anterior cervical diskectomy, the vertebral artery is at risk during lateral exploration of

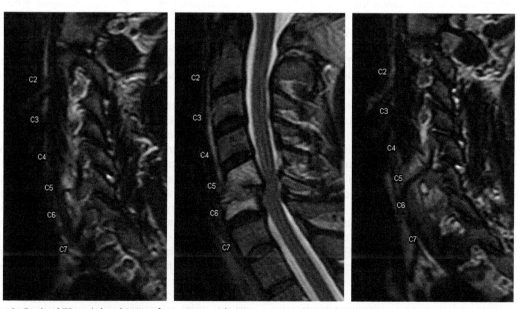

Fig. 4. Sagittal T2-weighted MRIs of a patient with C5/6 osteomyelitis/diskitis; right parasagittal (*left*), midsagittal (*middle*), and left parasagittal images (*right*) are shown. Note atypical left vertebral artery passage anterior to the C6 foramen and into the C5 foramen.

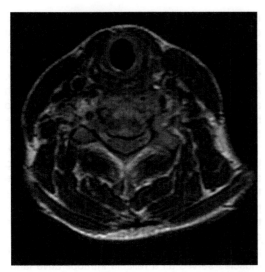

Fig. 5. Axial T2-weighted image of the same patient as in **Fig. 4** at the level of the inferior aspect of the C5 vertebral body demonstrating positioning of the left vertebral artery anterior to the vertebral foramina. A typical pattern is seen on the patient's right side.

the neural foramen. By limiting decompression laterally to the bony ridge of the uncovertebral joint, injury can generally be avoided. Removal of more laterally positioned osteophytes, however, can place the artery at risk, as can loss of orientation.[18]

When performing an anterior cervical corpectomy, the recommended width of decompression is approximately 16 mm.[21] Given that the average interforaminal distance varies from 26 mm to 29 mm, this amount of resection should be safe for nearly all patients at all vertebral levels. Excessive vertebral body resection laterally, however, can put the vertebral artery at risk. This can occur with asymmetric burring due to loss of midline orientation or as a result of oblique resection. The body wall opposite the side of surgical exposure is more prone to the latter, with the use of a surgical microscope considered a further risk factor for creating an oblique corpectomy trough. Additionally, the presence of a softened lateral cortex due to tumor or infection has been implicated in vertebral artery injury during corpectomy.[16–18]

Recommended strategies for avoidance of these complications include the use of multiple anatomic landmarks before and during decompression to assure safe resection. Prior to dissecting the longus colli, the midline can be marked using either a marking pen or electrocautery. Ensuring adequate visualization of the uncovertebral joints and planning a resection based on the use of a measuring standard of known width are important steps before beginning a corpectomy.

Once the decompression is started, further anatomic clues, such as the lateral curvature of the vertebral body, the location of epidural veins and fat, pedicle palpation, and visualization of the nerve roots, can all serve as verification of orientation.[16–18]

Lastly, the presence of a tortuous vertebral artery with erosion into the vertebral body can place the artery at risk despite strict adherence to the aforementioned principles.[11,19] Routine cervical MRI has been shown a reliable imaging modality for evaluation of this condition.[8] Studies have shown, however, that radiology reports of cervical spine MRIs often fail to comment on these and other vertebral artery anomalies and, therefore, all images should be scrutinized by an operating surgeon before any planned corpectomy or diskectomy.[22]

Should vertebral artery injury occur, options for management include tamponade, ligation, embolization, and repair. The therapeutic goals in treatment are 3-fold and progressive: (1) obtaining control of local hemorrhage, (2) prevention of immediate vertebrobasilar ischemia, and (3) prevention of cerebrovascular complications.

Initial tamponade should include the use of large pieces of hemostatic agents combined with pressure from surgical patties; this maneuver should be able to provide temporary hemostatis and can allow for anesthesia staff to obtain further vascular access. The use of particulate materials, such as bone wax, has been discouraged due to the theoretic risk of embolization. Because of the risk of postoperative hemorrhage, delayed embolic complications, and fistula or pseudoaneurysm formation, tamponade alone has largely been abandoned as definitive treatment.[17,23,24] Additionally, arterial ligature without prior visualization is not recommended due to the risk of nerve root damage.[16]

Once tamponade has provided some degree of hemostasis, resuscitation by the anesthesia staff should be performed before exposure of the vertebral artery for repair or ligation. Blood loss before obtaining temporary control is likely considerable, with reports ranging from 2300 mL to 4500 mL.[16] Exposure of the artery for repair or ligation is obtained by carrying dissection of the longus colli out further laterally over the transverse processes cephalad and caudad to the site of injury.[17] If the injury occurs ipsilateral to the side of exposure, this can be facilitated by various maneuvers. These include partial or complete transection of the sternocleidomastoid at the level of arterial injury, distal release of the sternocleidomastoid from its insertion site, and mobilization and retraction of the carotid sheath.[16]

Once exposed, transverse foramen can then be opened anteriorly by using either a high-speed burr or Kerrison rongeur. Additionally, the intertransversarii muscles covering the artery between the bones should be resected for improved exposure.[17] Clamps can be applied to the artery at this point for temporary control. Patency of the circle of Willis and adequate collateral circulation can be verified by noting continued bleeding through the site of arterial injury with maintenance of proximal clamping and simultaneous release of the distal clamp.[23] Surgical repair with the use of a 7-0 or 8-0 polypropylene suture has been recommended as the treatment of choice if possible, particularly when collateral circulation is not patent. Ligation, however, remains an option in patients with adequate collaterals.

The decision to ligate an injured vertebral artery is not without consequence. Although the vast majority of patients can tolerate unilateral vertebral artery ligation, in others it can lead to cerebellar or brainstem infarction. Patients with absence of a contralateral vertebral artery, a stenotic or hypoplastic contralateral vertebral artery, or inadequate collateralization at the circle of Willis are at risk of grave neurologic compromise with vertebral artery ligation. The reported incidence of left vertebral artery hypoplasia is 5.7% and the reported incidence of total absence of the left vertebral artery is 1.8%; these rates are 8.8% and 3.1% on the right. In patients without these anomalies, collateral flow can be compromised by atherosclerotic disease.[18] Overall mortality with unilateral vertebral artery ligation has been reported as high as 12%.[25] Other neurologic complications, such as Wallenberg syndrome, cerebellar infarction, isolated cranial nerve paresis, quadriparesis, and hemiplegia, have also been reported.

For these reasons, as well as the technical difficulty associated with open repair or ligation, angiography and coiling have been proposed as other treatment options, both acutely at the time of injury or with manifestation of late complications, such as pseudoaneurysm.[19,26] With angiography, the patency of collateral circulation can be definitively confirmed before embolization. This treatment option is dependent on the skill and availability of interventional providers at the time of injury, however, and only remains viable if patent collaterals exist.

In the few reported cases of vertebral artery injury during anterior spine surgery, a wide variety of outcomes exist. These vary from no significant neurologic or non-neurologic complications to cerebellar infarction to intraoperative exsanguination and death. In cases where a successful arterial repair was performed, none reports any long term neurologic or non-neurologic complications, making this the treatment of choice should injury occur.

SUBAXIAL POSTERIOR CERVICAL PROCEDURES

Posterior cervical procedures, including laminoplasty and foraminotomy, pose little risk to the vertebral artery. Posterior fixation techniques, namely, lateral mass and pedicle screw fixation for traumatic or postdecompression instability, place the vertebral artery at theoretic risk for injury, prompting inclusion in this discussion.

Many techniques for screw insertion have been described, with the Magerl technique the most frequently used.[27] When screws are laterally aimed in the axial plane, the vertebral artery, although not directly visualized by a surgeon, remains safe from injury. Large series on the complications of lateral mass screw fixation have been published without a report of vertebral artery injury.[28] No case reports of vertebral artery injury due to lateral mass screw placement exist in the literature.

Compared with lateral mass screws, subaxial cervical pedicle screws offer biomechanically improved fixation. The pedicles' anatomic position as the mdial wall of the transverse foramen, however, places the vertebral artery at risk in the event of a medial wall breach by a pedicle screw at a level where the vertebral artery passes through the transverse foramen. Although rare, vertebral artery injury with cervical pedicle screw placement has been reported.[29]

ATLANTOAXIAL FUSION

During posterior atlantoaxial fusion, the vertebral artery is at risk for injury during both exposure and placement of instrumentation. During exposure of the C1 ring posteriorly, the artery is relatively unprotected in the vertebral artery groove on the superior aspect of the arch. Injury can be avoided by limiting dissection to the inferior aspect of the C1 arch; additionally, the superior aspect of the arch can safely be dissected up to 8 mm from the midline.

Instrumentation techniques for atlantoaxial fusion have evolved significantly over time. Historically, posterior wiring procedures dominated but were subsequently replaced by Magerl transarticular screw fixation. The latter gained popularity due to the potential for spinal cord damage during sublaminar wire placement, offered a more rigid construct and significantly improved fusion rates over wiring.[30] The technique, however, placed the vertebral artery in significant peril, with published rates of vertebral artery injury as high as 8.2%.[31]

The ultimate goal of Magerl screw placement is safe screw passage through the C2 pars and into the lateral mass of C1. Prior to planning Magerl screw fixation, a surgeon must scrutinize cervical spine CT images for anomalous passage of the vertebral artery through the C2 lateral mass. Anatomic studies have shown that 20% of vertebrae have a vertebral artery course, which precludes safe passage of a 3.5-mm screw.[14] In patients with anatomy conducive to screw placement, vertebral artery injury can still occur at the inferior and lateral aspects of the safe zone. As a result, a trajectory passing through the most medial and dorsal aspects of the pars minimize the risk of vertebral artery injury.

Further identified risk factors for vertebral artery injury in patients with anatomy amenable to transarticular screw placement are (1) incomplete reduction before screw placement, (2) obliteration of the anterior tubercle of the atlas by prior transoral surgery, (3) failure to recognize an enlarged vertebral artery in the axis pedicle/lateral mass, and (4) damaged/deficient atlantoaxial lateral mass (eg, rheumatoid arthritis).[14,32]

For these and other reasons, C1/2 posterior screw/rod fixation (Harms) has gained considerable popularity over transarticular screw fixation. Although the vertebral artery remains at risk during both C2 pedicle and C1 lateral mass screw placement, these risks can be mitigated to a greater extent than with Magerl screw fixation. Intraoperative visualization of the C1 lateral mass screw entry point is key to proper screw placement but can be hampered by bleeding of the nearby venous plexus. Adequate hemostasis during this portion of the procedure is paramount, and risk of verterbral artery injury is lessened by the medial angulation of the C1 lateral mass screw by approximately 10°.[33]

Similar to transarticular screw placement, the risk of vertebral artery injury with the placement of a C2 pedicle screw can be minimized by accentuating medial and cephalad angulation during implant positioning. Although vertebral artery anomalies can preclude safe placement of segmental C2 fixation, this technique offers the flexibility bypassing that segment and extending the fusion to C3.[33]

Should vertebral artery injury occur during transarticular fixation or C2 instrumentation, the recommendation is to tamponade bleeding through screw placement or by using bone wax to fill the drilled hole. In these cases, angiography and coiling would are potentially useful postoperative adjuncts. If the artery is injured during exposure and can be visualized, direct repair is recommended.[32]

ILLUSTRATIVE CASE

A patient with multilevel cervical spondylotic myelopathy secondary to multilevel disease was consented for anterior cervical diskectomy and fusion at C4/5, C5/6, and C6/7. A standard Smith-Robinson anterior approach to the cervical spine was used with a left-sided, transverse incision. Operative level was verified using intraoperative radiograph. Dissection of longus colli muscles was performed using electrocautery; although dissection was being performed over the left C5/6 disk space, profuse bleeding was encountered from the superolateral region of the C6 body.

Because of the location and vigorousness of the bleeding, vertebral artery injury was suspected. Temporary hemostatis was obtained using thrombin-soaked gel foam and direct manual compression. This allowed time for placement of 2 large-bore IVs; additionally, blood products were brought to the operating room for hemodynamic support. At this point, the longus colli dissection was performed laterally to expose the vertebral artery as it entered into the C6 foramen. A 3-mm stellate laceration was noted within the artery wall (**Fig. 6**). Direct repair was attempted but was unsuccessful.

Proximal control was subsequently obtained via careful dissection through the longus colli caudad and exposure of the vertebral artery as it branched from the subclavian artery. Clamping of the artery at this point did not eliminate the hemorrhage, signifying patent collateral circulation but necessitating

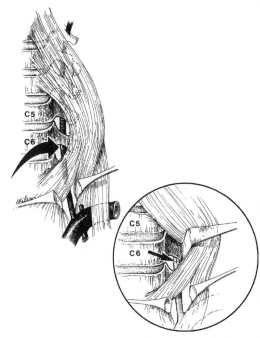

Fig. 6. Schematic demonstrating the vertebral artery passage into the C6 transverse foramen with left longus colli retracted laterally. Inset depicts stellate laceration visualized intraoperatively.

that distal control also be obtained. The remainder of the bony C6 foramen was exposed, and its anterior wall was removed using a Kerrison rongeur. This allowed for adequate distal arterial exposure to place a clamp, which controlled the bleeding. Because it was thought that the patient had adequate collateral circulation, the vertebral artery was ligated using silk ties and vascular hemoclips after another unsuccessful repair attempt (**Fig. 7**).

The previously intended diskectomies were subsequently performed with a final operative blood loss of 2 L. Somatosensory evoked potentials remained unchanged throughout the case, and the patient had no new neurologic deficits postoperatively.

OESPHOGEAL ANATOMY

The pharynx and esophagus are deep, thin-walled, cervical viscera. The hypopharynx is the portion of the digestive tract, which spans from the hyoid bone to the inferior border of the cricoid cartilage. It connects with the trachea ventrally and esophagus dorsally; the latter connection occurs at the level of the C6 vertebra. The esophagus itself is 23 cm to 25 cm in length and travels along the anterior aspect of the vertebral column, through the superior and posterior mediastinum as well as through the diaphragm. It terminates in the cardiac orifice of the stomach, opposite the eleventh thoracic vertebrae. With the cervical spine,

it resides posterior to the trachea and anterior to the longus colli muscles; in anterior spine procedures, it is retracted medially along with the other midline cervical structures (**Fig. 8**).

The region of the esophagus most at risk for perforation with instrumentation is the cricopharyngeal region of the cervical esophagus. Termed, *Lannier's triangle*, this region is bordered by the constrictor pharyngeus and cricopharyngeus muscles at the level of the C5/6. In this area, the posterior esophageal mucosa is covered only by a thin fascial layer, making injury by instrumentation or anterior vertebral osteophytes more likely.[34]

CAUSES AND INCIDENCE

Esophageal injury during anterior cervical spine procedures is a rare occurrence, with reported rates that range from 0.3% in elective cervical diskectomy and fusion to 1.49% in cases of cervical spine trauma and 1.6% in cervical corpectomy cases.[35–37] Acute injuries can be caused during sharp surgical dissection, by inappropriately placed retractor blades, by a direct surgical injury, or by a traumatic endotracheal intubation.[38] Additionally, perforations can occur with blunt or penetrating trauma, accounting for the increased incidence seen within this patient population.

The additional subset of patients with iatrogenic esophageal injury after anterior spine surgery can be directly attributed to instrumentation, namely

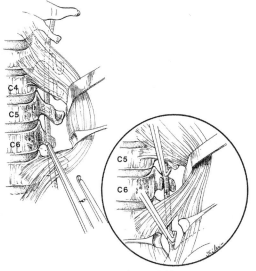

Fig. 7. Schematic depicting the exposure of the vertebral artery within the C6 foramen using a Kerrison rongeur. Inset demonstrates the obtaining of proximal and distal hemostasis with temporary clamps to allow for definitive treatment.

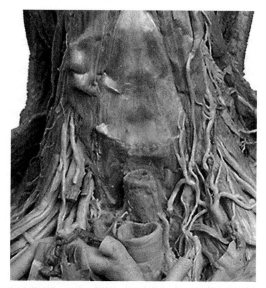

Fig. 8. Gross specimen depicting the relationship between the cervical spinal column, esophagus, and trachea.

anterior plating systems. Prior to the advent of these systems, large case series of anterior spine procedures reported on by Cloward,[39] and subsequently Barber,[40] had no reported cases of esophageal injury. Late presentation after anterior screw migration,[41–43] overt instrumentation failure,[44] or instrumented anterior fusion with no evidence of instrumentation failure[45] have all subsequently been reported. As a result, the true incidence of these complications is difficult to quantify.

PRESENTATION AND DIAGNOSIS

The presentation of a patient esophageal injury and subsequent diagnosis thereof is largely dependent on the timing relative to surgery when suspicion for injury is raised. Concern for acute intraoperative injury should prompt visual inspection of the esophagus. Intraesophageal dye injection has been suggested as an adjunct for diagnosing acute injury when suspicion exists but no obvious rent is visible.[46]

When an acute injury occurs but is not noted intraoperatively, patients generally present in the early postoperative phase. Signs and symptoms concerning for esophageal injury include dysphagia, odynophagia, subcutaneous emphysema, neck swelling, dyspnea, and fever. The presence of swallowed food draining from the operative wound is considered pathognomonic for esophageal injury, and patients may also present with cervical abscess or overt septicemia.[35,36,47,48]

Late perforation caused by instrumentation or graft erosion into the esophagus can occur months to years after the index procedure. These patients present in a more varied manner, which can range from that in the early postoperative presentation (described previously) or with other, more subtle findings, such as recurrent pneumonia, fevers, neck pain, and dysphagia.[41,43,49] Presentation can also be less subtle with oral or rectal passage of loosened instrumentation.

A variety of laboratory studies and imaging modalities have been shown useful in diagnosing esophageal injury. In the presence of infection or abscess, inflammatory markers, such as C-reactive protein and erythrocyte sedimentation rate, are markedly elevated. Plain radiography can demonstrate gross loosening of instrumentation. CT scan can demonstrate prevertebral air, whereas MRI can show cervical abscess or osteomyelitis. Barium swallow evaluations with gross extravasation of contrast verify the diagnosis, as does visualization of a defect on upper endoscopy.[36,47,48,50]

Further complications seen after esophageal perforation are numerous and significant. These include wound breakdown, malnutrition, osteomyelitis, pneumonia, mediastinitis, acute respiratory distress syndrome, sepsis, and death.[51] Infectious organsims implicated in these cases include streptococcus, Staphylococcus aureus, pseudomonas, bacteroides, anaerobic gram-positive cocci, and candida albicans.[52]

TREATMENT

When a direct esophageal injury occurs and is noted intraoperatively, direct repair at the time of surgery with absorbable suture is indicated. Intraoperative placement of a nasogastric tube, drain, and standard closure should follow. The patient should be treated with broad-spectrum antibiotics, continuous saliva suctioning, and enteral feeding via the nasogastric tube. Nasogastric feeding is continued for approximately 10 days and oral feeding is initiated after a barium swallow study with no evidence of extravasation and endoscopy, with no visible defect noted. If the injury occurs and is noted during exposure, any planned diskectomy/corpectomy should be abandoned and performed on a delayed basis once the esophageal rent is fully healed. Outcomes from this type of injury and treatment are reported as universally excellent with no long-term sequelae.[47,51]

With early and late postoperative presentation, initial treatment includes wound exploration. Removal of instrumentation may or may not be appropriate based on the clinical situation. The esophagus should be inspected for a defect, with primary closure performed if possible. Extensive débridements may be necessary, including débridement of cervical abscess, osteomyelitis, and mediastinitis via thoracotomy, as appropriate. Esophageal stenting with salivary bypass tubes and sternocleidomastoid muscle flaps have been advocated as an adjunct to repair. Wound management can either be primary closure over drains or open wound care, with the latter reported to have a higher infectious cure rate. Postoperative care includes enteral feeding via a nasogastric tube, continuous saliva suctioning, and broad-spectrum antibiotics with repeat débridements, as necessary. These treatments are continued until full healing has occurred as evidenced by esophogram with no extravasation and endoscopy with no visible perforation.[47,51–53]

Outcomes are varied because of the spectrum of complications that can be seen with esophageal injury. Hospitalizations for this condition have been reported to range from 13 to 213 days, with median ICU stays of 10 days. Mortality rates range from 20% to 50%, with aggressive, early intervention considered the best opportunity for a good outcome. For this reason, historically espoused conservative management has largely fallen out of favor.[47,51,52]

ILLUSTRATIVE CASE

A 53-year-old woman was diagnosed with cervical spondylotic myelopathy and treated with an uncomplicated C5 and C6 corpectomy, C4 to C7 anterior fusion with fibular allograft and instrumentation (**Fig. 9**). On postoperative day 3, the patient developed worsening dysphagia, stridor, neck pain, and fevers; on presentation to the emergency department, CT scan was performed and the patient was diagnosed with a cervical abscess (**Fig. 10**) and associated mediastinitis (**Fig. 11**). She underwent emergent drainage of abscess with tracheostomy placement. A perforation of the posterior pharyngeal wall above the cricopharyngeus was noted and primarily repaired. Her surgical wound was closed over a 10-mm

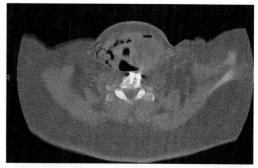

Fig. 10. Cervical CT demonstrating large cervical abscess with compression and lateral deviation of the trachea.

Jackson-Pratt drain. She concominantly underwent a thorascopic mediastinal irrigation and débridement with drain placement. Postoperatively, she was placed on broad-spectrum antibiotics and defervesced. Three days later, she developed confusion, fevers, and increasing white blood cell count; a follow-up CT was performed and demonstrated an anterior mediastinal collection. This was treated with a débridement via an anterior thoracotomy and second rib removal. Postoperatively, the patient tolerated enteral tube feeds, and serial barium swallow studies were performed until no extravasation was seen (**Fig. 12**). She was transferred out of the ICU on hospital day 9 and eventually discharged to home on normal enteral feeds on hospital day 17 (**Fig. 13**).

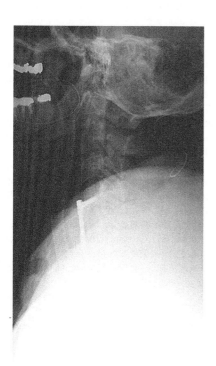

Fig. 9. Intraoperative film after C4-C7 anterior cervical corpectomy and fusion demonstrating instrumentation in good position.

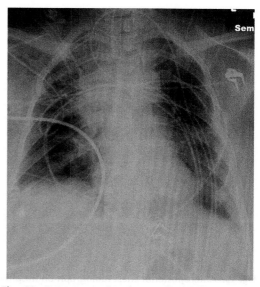

Fig. 11. Anteroposterior chest radiograph consistent with mediastinitis.

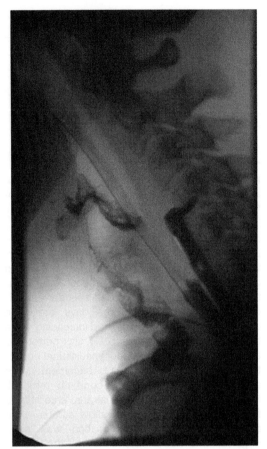

Fig. 12. Initial barium swallow study performed on hospital day 9, demonstrating contrast extravasation.

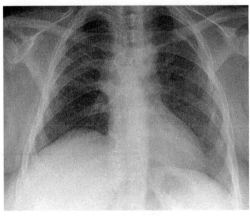

Fig. 13. Anteroposterior chest radiograph on hospital day 17, just before discharge, demonstrating resolution of mediastinitis.

REFERENCES

1. Moore KL, Dally AF. Clinically oriented anatomy. 4th edition. Philadelphia: Lippincott, Williams & Wilkens; 1999.
2. Heary RF, Albert TJ, Ludwig SC, et al. Surgical anatomy of the vertebral arteries. Spine 1996;18: 2074–80.
3. Bohlman HH. Cervical spondylosis with moderate to severe myelopathy: a report of seventeen cases treated by Robinson anterior cervical discectomy and fusion. Spine 1997;2:151–62.
4. Vaccaro AR, Ring D, Scuderi F, et al. Vertebral artery location in relation to the vertebral body as determined by two-dimensional computed tomography evaluation. Spine 1994;19:2637–41.
5. Pushchak TJ, Vaccaro AR, Rauschning W, et al. Relevant surgical anatomy of the cervical, thoracic, and lumbar spine. In: Betz RR, Zeidman SM, editors. Priniciples and practice of spine surgery. Philadelphia: Mosby; 2003.
6. Madawi AA, Solanki G, Casey ATH, et al. Variation of the groove in the axis vertebra for the vertebral artery: impications for instrumentation. J Bone Joint Surg Br 1997;79:820–3.
7. Ebraheim NA, Xu R, Ahmad M, et al. The quantitative anatomy of the vertebral artery groove of the atlas and its relation to the posterior atlantoaxial approach. Spine 1998;23:320–3.
8. Eskander MS, Drew JM, Aubin ME, et al. Vertebral artery anatomy: a review of two hundred fifty magnetic resonance imaging scans. Spine 2010; 35:2035–40.
9. Slover WP, Kiley RF. Cervical vertebral erosion caused by tortuous vertebral artery. Radiology 1995;84:112–4.
10. Lindsey RW, Piepmeier J, Burkus JK. Tortuosity of the vertebral artery: an adventitious finding after cervical trauma. J Bone Joint Surg 1985;67:806–8.
11. Tumialan LM, Wippold FJ, Morgan RA. Tortuous vertebral artery injury complicating anterior cervical spinal fusion in a symptomatic rheumatoid cervical spine. Spine 2004;29:E343–8.
12. Curylo LJ, Mason HC, Bohlman HH, et al. Tortuous course of the vertebral artery and anterior spinal decompression: a cadaveric and clinical case study. Spine 2002;25:2860–4.
13. Hong JT, Park DK, Lee MJ, et al. Anatomical variations of the vertebral artery segment in the lower cervical spine: analysis by three-dimensional computed tomography angiography. Spine 2008;33:2422–6.
14. Madawi AA, Casey A, Solanki G, et al. Radiological and anatomical evaluation of the atlantoaxial transarticular screw fixation technique. Neurosurgery 1997; 86:961–8.
15. Young JP, Young PH, Ackerman MJ, et al. The ponticulus posticus: Implications for screw insertion into

the first cervical lateral mass. J Bone Joint Surg Am 2005;87:2495–8.

16. Smith MD, Emery SE, Dudley A, et al. Vertebral artery injury during anterior decompression of the cervical spine: a retrospective review of ten patients. J Bone Joint Surg Br 1993;75:410–5.

17. Golfinos JG, Dickman CA, Zabramski JM, et al. Repair of vertebral artery injury during anterior cervical decompression. Spine 1994;12:2552–6.

18. Burke JP, Gerszten PC, Welch WC. Iatrogenic vertebral artery injury during anterior cervical spine surgery. Spine J 2005;5:508–14.

19. Eskander MS, Connolly PJ, Eskander JP, et al. Injury of an aberrant vertebral artery during a routine corpectomy: a case report and literature review. Spinal Cord 2009;47:773–5.

20. Bae HW, Delamarter RB. Cervical vertebrectomy and plating. In: Zdeblick TA, Bradford DS, editors. Masters techniques in orthopaedic surgery: the spine. Philadelphia: Lippincott, Williams & Wilkens; 2004. p. 47–66.

21. Farmer JC. Anterior cervical corpectomy. In: Abert TJ, Vaccaro AR, editors. Spine surgery: tricks of the trade. 2nd edition. New York: Thieme Medical Publishers; 2009. p. 62–4.

22. Aubin ME, Eskander MS, Drew JM, et al. Indentification of type 1 interforaminal vertebral artery anomalies in cervical spine MRI's. Spine 2010;35: E1610–1.

23. Pfeifer BA, Friedberg SR, Jewell ER. Repair of injured vertebral artery in anterior cervical procedures. Spine 1994;19:1471–4.

24. Golueke P, Sclafani S, Phillips T, et al. Vertebral artery injury: diagnosis and management. J Trauma 1987; 27:856–65.

25. Shintani A, Zervas NT. Consequence of ligation of the vertebral artery. Neurosurgery 1972;36: 447–50.

26. Choi JW, Lee JK, Moon KS, et al. Endovascular embolization of iatrogenic vertebral artery injury during anterior cervical spine surgery: a report of two cases and review of the literature. Spine 2006; 31:E891–4.

27. Ebraheim N. Posterior lateral mass screw fixation: anatomic and radiographic considerations. Univ Penn Ortho J 1999;12:66–72.

28. Heller JG, Silcox H, Sutterlin CE. Complications of posterior cervical plating. Spine 1995;20: 2442–8.

29. Abumi K, Shono Y, Ito M, et al. Complications of pedicle screw fixation in reconstructive surgery of the cervical spine. Spine 2000;25: 962–9.

30. Jeanneret B, Magerl F. Primary posterior C1/2 fusion in odontoid fractures: Indications, technique, and results of transarticular screw fixation. J Spinal Disord 1992;5:464–75.

31. Neo M, Fujibayashi S, Miyata M, et al. Vertebral artery injury during cervical spine surgery. Spine 2008;33:779–85.

32. Peng CW, Chou BT, Bendo JA, et al. Vertebral artery injury in cervical spine surgery: anatomical considerations, management, and preventative measures. Spine J 2009;9:70–6.

33. Harms J, Melcher RP. Posterior C1-C2 fusion with polyaxial screw and rod fixation. Spine 2001;26: 2467–71.

34. Jones WG, Ginsberg RJ. Esophageal perforation: a continuing challenge. Ann Thorac Surg 1992;53: 534–43.

35. Fountas KN, Kapsalaki EZ, Nikolakakos LG, et al. Anterior cervical discectomy and fusion associated complications. Spine 2007;32:2310–7.

36. Gaudinez RF, English GM, Gebhard JS, et al. Esophageal perforations after anterior cervical surgery. J Spinal Disord 2000;13:77–84.

37. Elaraky MA, Llanos C, Sonntag VK. Cervical corpectomy: report of 185 cases and review of the literature. J Neurosurg 1999;90:25–41.

38. Levine PA. Hypopharingeal perforation: an untoward complication of endotracheal intubation. Arch Surg 1979;111:578–80.

39. Cloward RB. Complications of anterior cervical disk operation and their treatment. Surgery 1971; 69:175–82.

40. Barber FA. Anterior cervical fusion: the postoperative complications. Rocky Mt Med J 1978;75: 29–33.

41. Sahjpaul RL. Esophageal perforation from anterior cervical screw migration. Surg Neurol 2007;68: 205–10.

42. Smith MD, Bolesta MJ. Esophageal perforation after anterior cervical plate fixation: a report of two cases. J Spinal Disord 1992;5:357–62.

43. Hanci M, Toprak M, Sarioglu AC, et al. Oesophageal perforation subsequent to anterior cervical spine screw/plate fixation. Paraplegia 1995;33:606–9.

44. Fujibayashi S, Shikata J, Kamiya N, et al. Missing anterior cervical plate and screws: a case report. Spine 2000;25:2258–61.

45. Witwer BP, Resnick DK. Delayed esophageal injury without instrumentation failure: complication of anterior cervical instrumentation. J Spinal Disord Tech 2003;16:519–23.

46. Taylor B, Patel AA, Okubadejo GO, et al. Detection of esophageal perforation using intraesophageal dye injection. J Spinal Disord Tech 2006;19:191–3.

47. Orlando ER, Caroli E, Ferrante L. Management of the cervical esophagus and hypofarinx perforations complicating anterior cervical spine surgery. Spine 2003;28:E290–5.

48. Patel NP, Wolcott WP, Johnson JP, et al. Esophageal injury associated with anterior cervical spine surgery. Surg Neurol 2008;69:20–4.

49. Lu DC, Theodore P, Korn WM, et al. Esophageal erosion 9 years after anterior cervical plate implantation. Surg Neurol 2008;69:310–3.

50. Mattingly WT, Dillon ML, Todd EP. Cervical osteomyelitis after esophageal perforation. South Med J 1982;75:626–7.

51. Newhouse KE, Lindsey RW, Clark CR, et al. Esophageal perforation following anterior spine surgery. Spine 1989;14:1051–3.

52. Rueth N, Shaw D, Groth S, et al. Management of cervical esophageal injury after spinal surgery. Ann Thorac Surg 2010;90:1128–33.

53. Benazzo M, Spasiano R, Bertino G, et al. Sternocleidomastoid muscle flap in esophageal perforation repair after cervical spine surgery: concepts, techniques, and personal experience. J Spinal Disord Tech 2008;21:597–605.

Diagnosis and Management of Metastatic Cervical Spine Tumors

Camilo A. Molina, BA, Ziya L. Gokaslan, MD,
Daniel M. Sciubba, MD*

KEYWORDS

- Cervical spine tumors • Metastasis • Palliative therapy
- Vertebrectomy

The skeletal system is the third most common site after the lungs and liver for distant cancer metastasis regardless of primary tumor pathology. Within the skeletal system, the bony spine is the most commonly affected site, with approximately 33% of cancer patients developing metastatic spine lesions.[1] However, despite the bony spine being the most common site of osseous involvement for patients with metastatic cancer, the cervical spine is only involved in 8% to 20% of metastatic spine disease cases.[2] Nonetheless, given the 1.5 million newly diagnosed cases of cancer annually,[3] encountering metastatic lesions within the cervical spine is not of rare occurrence.

The initial approach to diagnosis and management of cervical spine tumors requires an organizational framework that categorizes a presentation according to the compartment involved, the pathology of the lesion, and the anatomic region involved. The compartment involved refers to whether the lesion is located in the epidural, intradural-extramedullary, or intramedullary compartment, and is essential in not only formulating an initial differential diagnosis but also in understanding the pathophysiology of the lesion as it pertains to patient presenting signs and symptoms.[4,5] The pathology of the lesion is of utmost importance, as it has the largest role in dictating management. For example, if a lesion is of primary rather than metastatic origin, then a curative surgical intervention (ie, en bloc resection)[6] is a possibility, whereas surgical intervention in the setting of a metastatic lesion may only serve a palliative role given that the patient is most likely also concomitantly afflicted with numerous systemic lesions.[7–10] The anatomic region involved is divided into 3 component regions: the craniovertebral junction (CVJ; C0–C1), subaxial spine (C3–C7), and the cervicothoracic junction (C7–T1). Each of these component regions has unique biomechanical properties, thereby influencing management decisions. For example, the surgical approach to achieving en bloc resection of a tumor affecting the CVJ is very different from the approach if the same lesion is located within the subaxial spine. This article describes the diagnosis and management of metastatic epidural cervical spine tumors based on the latter considerations.

EPIDEMIOLOGY

Although the thoracic spine is most commonly occupied by metastatic lesions, the cervical spine harbors metastatic lesions in 8% to 20% of cases.[11] It is thought that the wide range in the reported incidence of cervical spine affliction is attributable to whether asymptomatic or symptomatic involvement is reported.[11] The most common primary tumor pathologies are breast, prostate, and non–small cell lung carcinoma.[12] The highest incidence of spinal metastases occurs among individuals in the fourth and sixth decade, and men are more likely to be afflicted than women.[5] There are several mechanisms by which a primary neoplasm

Department of Neurosurgery, Johns Hopkins University, 600 North Wolfe Street, Baltimore, MD 21287, USA
* Corresponding author. 600 North Wolfe Street, Meyer 5-185a, Baltimore, MD.
E-mail address: dsciubb1@jhmi.edu

Orthop Clin N Am 43 (2012) 75–87
doi:10.1016/j.ocl.2011.08.004
0030-5898/12/$ – see front matter © 2012 Elsevier Inc. All rights reserved.

can metastasize to the spine, with the mechanism depending on primary tumor pathology. Tumor pathology dictates primary tumor location and biological behavior, both of which are factors that influence spread mechanisms. Specifically, the 3 main mechanisms by which a lesion can metastasize to the spine are direct extension or invasion, hematogenous metastasis, and cerebrospinal fluid (CSF) seeding. Direct invasion or extension occurs through primary lesions becoming locally aggressive and extending to involve the bony spine. Hematogenous seeding is facilitated by the vast arterial supply of the vertebrae and via the valveless venous drainage plexi such as Batson's plexus. Seeding of a primary lesion through the CSF occurs much less frequently and is most often caused by surgical manipulation of primary or metastatic cerebral lesions.[13] A retrospective study by Chaichana and colleagues[7] found that among lesions originating from breast, kidney, lung, gastrointestinal, and prostate cancers; breast metastatic lesions were the only ones found to have a statistically significant predisposition to metastasize to the cervical spine.

PRESENTATION

Metastatic disease to the cervical spine can present with a variety of clinical signs and symptoms[11]; however, it is also not uncommon to detect asymptomatic cervical metastasis when working up an unrelated problem.[11,14] Presenting symptoms include mechanical, nonmechanical, and referred pain due to pathologic fracture; as well as neurologic dysfunction due to spinal cord or nerve root compression.[2,11,12,15,16] The most common presenting symptom with metastatic cervical lesions is localized nonmechanical pain, present in approximately 89% to 93% of patients.[1,11,12,16,17] This pain is often described as not being related to any activities, progressively worsening, and exacerbated in the evening. Furthermore, the pain can be either unilateral or bilateral as well as either focal or referred. When referred, the pain often radiates to the shoulder and trapezial area. It is important to suspect and rule out the presence of metastatic disease in the setting of a patient with a previous history of carcinoma and a new onset of nonmechanical pain.[4,17,18]

The next most common presenting symptom is mechanical pain.[4] This type of pain is relieved by rest and/or stabilization and is exacerbated by motion. As in the thoracic and lumbar segments, the vertebral body of a cervical vertebra is the primary site of seeding of metastatic deposits. Lytic or erosive lesions of local cancellous bone thereby increase the risk of pathologic collapse.[11]

Due to the greater proportion of cancellous bone in the subaxial spine, the presentation of mechanical pain varies according to whether the lesion involves the atlantoaxial or subaxial spine. Collapse within the subaxial spine may lead to an angular kyphotic deformity resulting in mechanical pain and/or neurologic dysfunction. Unlike the subaxial spine, metastatic spread to the CVJ is rare, only accounting for 0.5% of all metastatic spine lesions.[19,20] Given the anatomic uniqueness of the CVJ, cancellous bone destruction in the CVJ does not result in as much angular kyphosis and flexion/extension instability as in the subaxial spine. Instead, the biomechanical instability of the upper cervical spine is dependent on an intact transverse ligament and lateral articular masses. More commonly, destruction of the lateral masses results in painful rotational instability, and destruction of the C2 spinous processes accompanied by detachment of the paraspinal musculature often manifests as patients complaining of an inability to hold the head upright unassisted.[21]

Neurologic dysfunction is the next most common presenting complaint, occurring in approximately 5% to 10% of patients.[4] Cervical radiculopathy most commonly occurs as a result of foraminal invasion by the tumor and presents as a burning, dyesthetic type of pain. Long tract signs are the next most common and include atrophy of intrinsic hand muscles, ambulation difficulty, myelopathic hand syndrome, and extremity spasticity. Autonomic dysfunction such as sphincter disturbance is the least common, often being a late finding that indicates advanced disease and thus a poor prognosis for neurologic function recovery.[21,22] In general, spinal cord compression occurs more commonly in the subaxial area for several reasons. First, tumor or retropulsed bone invading the anterior epidural space is more common with tumor in the subaxial spine vertebral bodies. Second, there is a relatively larger spinal canal in the atlantoaxial region compared with the subaxial spine, so lesions can grow larger at the craniocervical junction prior to spinal cord compression. Finally, the complex of craniocervical ligaments often serves as a barrier to invasion of the canal by ventrally situated tumors. In the subaxial spine, the only barrier is the diminutive posterior longitudinal ligament.

DIAGNOSIS

Any patient with a known history of cancer presenting with persistent neck pain (including mechanical and nonmechanical) should be evaluated for a metastatic pathologic process. In addition, any patient with persistent nonmechanical pain should also receive evaluation for a neoplastic process involving the cervical spine.[11] Physical examination is an essential part of the primary workup and should be performed meticulously to elicit important findings such as palpable masses, pain, and neurologic dysfunction—including both motor and sensory loss. The type of pain elicited can help localize the location of the lesion. Pain elicited on flexion/extension more commonly corresponds to lesions localized to the subaxial spine, whereas pain elicited on rotational motion more commonly corresponds to lesions involving the CVJ.[12] In addition, a history of nocturnal pain and an ability to elicit local pain on applied pressure further increases the suspicion of a neoplastic process.

Early recognition of neurologic dysfunction is important, as pre-operative neurologic function is the most positive prognostic factor for postintervention neurologic status.[23] Common signs of neurologic deficit include spasticity, hyperreflexia, paraparesis, Hoffman sign, abnormal plantar responses, and occasionally Brown-Sequard syndrome. Because tumors localized to the CVJ have a decreased incidence of neurologic manifestations due to the wider canal space of the CVJ, neurologic deficits are more often caused by antlantoaxial subluxation rather than direct cord compression. Lastly, cerebellar ataxia may occur if the neoplasm extends across the foramen magnum.[24]

Following physical examination, imaging is the next most important step in the diagnostic workup and should include plain radiographs, magnetic resonance imaging (MRI), computed tomography (CT), and bone scintigraphy.[11] Plain radiographs permit assessment of spinal stability, the location and extent of metastatic lesions, and evaluation of the disk space.[11] Signs of spinal instability include progressive deformity, significant translation or angulation, and/or greater than 50% involvement of the vertebral body. Lesions are evidenced by a variety of destructive changes such as spinous process erosion, vertebral body osteolysis, and an inability to visualize the pedicle. In addition, elevation of soft-tissue shadows may also be observed.[11] Cervical disk spaces in the setting of metastatic spine disease are well maintained unless the neoplastic process has resulted in pathologic collapse, in which case the space will be narrowed.[11] Unfortunately, plain radiographs lack sensitivity in detecting lesions, as plain radiographs typically cannot detect lesions until 30% to 50% of the bone is demineralized.

The gold-standard imaging modality is MRI given its exceptional ability to visualize the bone-soft tissue interface, resulting in a highly detailed rendition of compression and/or invasion of osseous, neural, and paraspinal structures.[4,11] For example,

T2-weighted MRI can provide direct evidence of cord compression and the degree of spinal stenosis (**Fig. 1**). Osseous invasion can be visualized as the replacement of normal marrow fat signal with neoplastic tissue. Specifically, bone marrow signal in tumor and infection shows increased and decreased intensity on T2-weighted and T1-weighted imaging, respectively. Furthermore, the use of gadolinium on T1-weighted imaging may further enhance visualization of marrow invasion by tumor tissue.[25,26]

CT imaging is complementary to MRI in detecting and evaluating lesions, as it provides exceptional rendition detail of the bony spine, spinal canal, and any osseous compressive structures such as retropulsed bony fragments following pathologic collapse. Furthermore, CT with myelography is the gold-standard imaging modality for patients who have contraindications to MRI.[12,27]

Of note, only 11% of metastatic cervical neoplasms are isolated lesions, with lesions also commonly occurring in both the axial and appendicular skeleton.[14] Bone scintigraphy therefore may be used as a method for conducting a screen in search of additional metastatic lesions localizing to the skeletal system. Furthermore, bone scintigraphy is also an excellent modality to screen for

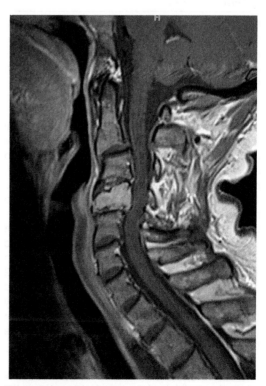

Fig. 1. T1-weighted magnetic resonance image showing relation of metastatic spine tumor to spinal cord.

possible bony metastatic lesions in high-risk patients (ie, patients with a history of prostate cancer). However, it must be remembered that bone scintigraphy is a measure of bone turnover, and findings are not specific to a neoplastic process and may be due to healing fractures, spondylosis, or infection—therefore, findings should always be confirmed by MRI or CT. Furthermore, bone scintigraphy cannot provide a detailed rendition of bony anatomy nor provide any information on the extent of cord compression.[24,28]

Biopsy sampling establishes a histopathologic diagnosis and is essential in determining the surgical strategy and tumor stage. At the cervical level, an anterolateral approach with fine-needle aspiration under CT guidance can be performed to obtain a sample of the tissue in question.[4,11]

MANAGEMENT

Optimal management of metastatic cervical spine disease requires a multidisciplinary approach including, but not limited to, medical, surgical, and radiation oncology cooperation. Treatment options range from palliative nonoperative treatment to aggressive surgical intervention; therefore, appropriate patient selection for a particular treatment modality is a crucial component of management.

Patient Selection

Patients' characteristics such as age, medical history, current medical condition, and overall life expectancy must be considered when constructing a management plan. Although age is not an absolute contraindication to surgical management, a patient's age must be considered in the context of systemic cancer disease and comorbid medical conditions to estimate an individual patient's life expectancy and to assess whether that expectancy is sufficiently long enough to benefit from surgical intervention. Specifically, patients with a life expectancy of less than 8 to 12 weeks are generally more apt to undergo nonoperative management. Accurate determination of tumor pathology is also essential in patient selection, as it is the most significant prognostic factor for survival.[4,11,29] For example, median survival of a metastatic bony lung tumor is 7 to 9 months whereas median survival for metastatic bony breast neoplasms is 30 months.[11] A study conducted by Rao and colleagues[14] found that the mean survival for all metastatic tumors to the bony cervical spine was 14.7 months.

Various classification systems have been published to objectively assess which patients are adequate candidates for surgical intervention in the setting of metastatic spine disease. Harrington[30] classifies patients according to the degree of bony and neurologic compromise. Kostuik and colleagues[31] assessed the necessity of surgical intervention based on the lesions' likelihood of resulting in mechanical instability. DeWald and colleagues[32] developed a system similar to that of both Harrington and colleagues and Kostuik and colleagues, with the additional component of scoring the immunocompetence of each patient. Tokuhashi and colleagues[29] devised a system that not only assesses the pathology of the lesion in question but also considers additional spinal and extraspinal metastasis, as well as overall patient condition, neurologic status, and primary tumor pathology. Ultimately, regardless of which system is used, the practitioner must carefully weigh the risks and benefits for each individual patient when considering whether to offer surgical intervention.

Staging

Once a patient has been selected to undergo surgical management, determining the extent of surgical management (ie, palliative vs curative) requires staging of the lesion on the vertebral arch[33] and the extent of paraspinal structure involvement.[34] Various staging systems have been devised to determine the best form of therapeutic option (**Table 1**). The main purpose of each system is to recommend whether a particular lesion is amenable to curative (ie, total vertebrectomy) versus palliative (ie, decompressive or debulking) surgical intervention. Of note, the scoring system proposed by Tokuhashi and colleagues[29,35] allows for not only patient selection but also for planning the extent of surgical management.

Nonoperative Management

In general, nonsurgical management of metastatic spine disease is recommended when tumor involvement has not resulted in any of the following: (1) spinal instability, (2) neurologic deficit, and (3) pain nonresponsive to medical management.[16]

Nonsurgical management includes radiotherapy, chemotherapy, hormonal therapy, and high-dose steroid therapy. Radiation therapy is most appropriate in the setting of the aforementioned indications. Additional indications for radiation therapy include the presence of multiple noncontiguous lesions affecting the bony spine and the caveat that the patient must not have been treated by this method before.[11] The response to radiation therapy varies by tumor type, with prostate and breast tumor generally being more radiosensitive than renal and lung tumors.[36–38] Positive response to tumor therapy can be measured by decreased tumor size and local pain.[36,37,39–41]

Table 1
Staging and scoring systems proposed to plan intervention

	Rationale	Method	Recommendation
Tomita Scoring System[34]	Provides anatomic description of tumor extension within vertebrae and paravertebral tissues	Vertebrae divided into 7 sites: 1. Vertebral body 2. Pedicle 3. Lamina and spinous process 4. Spinal canal (epidural space) 5. Paravertebral area 6. Adjacent vertebrae 7. Multiple skip lesions	Total en bloc spondylectomy recommended for type 2, 3, 4, and 5 lesions Relatively indicated for type 1 and 6 lesions Contraindicated for type 7 lesions
Weinstein-Boriani-Biagini Staging System[82]	Precise data-gathering tool to describe tumor involvement of vertebral body and adjacent tissues	Vertebrae divided into 12 sectors in clock-face arrangement beginning at the spinous process Five tissue layers are defined: a. Extraosseous soft tissues b. Intraosseous superficial c. Intraosseous deep d. Extraosseous extradural e. Extraosseous intradural	Tumor description using this system allows surgeon to plan surgery and gather data uniformly. Particularly useful in describing tumor involvement to other practitioners
Tokuhashi Scoring System[35]	Considers extraspinal tumor involvement and overall condition to estimate patient prognosis and guide treatment	Six parameters used with respective score assigned: 1. General condition 2. Number of extraspinal bone metastases 3. Number of metastases in vertebral body 4. Metastases to major internal organs 5. Primary site of cancer 6. Palsy	All categories range from 0 to 2 points with exception of primary tumor pathology (5 points maximum), placing highest prognostic weight on primary tumor site Score recommendation: <8 (<6 mo survival): nonoperative or palliative treatment 9–11 (>6 mo survival): palliative surgery or excisional surgery if single lesion and no extraspinal metastases 12–15 (≥1 year survival): excisional surgery

Various optimal radiation-dose protocols have been proposed, but to date randomized control trials have not elucidated an optimal dosing regimen. Kaasa and colleagues,[42] Nielsen and colleagues,[43] and Maranzano and colleagues[44] performed randomized controlled trials to evaluate comparative efficacies of single-dose versus fractionated-dose radiation therapy, and failed to find statistically significant differences in pain, functional, and complication outcomes.

Although radiation therapy as a primary management modality may be adequate in the absence of spinal instability and neurologic deficit, the efficacy of radiation therapy as a primary management modality in the setting of neurologic deficit without spinal instability versus that of surgical intervention has been a point of controversy. In 2005, Patchell and colleagues[45] conducted a randomized controlled trial comparing the relative efficacy of surgery alone, radiotherapy alone, and radiotherapy and surgery combined. The group determined that both survival and functional outcomes were superior in the group undergoing both surgical and radiation therapy.

Novel stereotactic radiosurgery techniques have the advantage of delivery of high-intensity radiation with consistent precision and increased accuracy, permitting the delivery of higher doses while minimizing damage of adjacent radiosensitive structures. However, there are currently no randomized controlled studies that demonstrate a superior efficacy of this method to that of conventional radiation therapy. Nonetheless, current evidence indicates that radiosurgery is an efficacious management option. Wowra and colleagues[41] conducted a prospective case series study (Class II evidence) with the objective of assessing the clinical results of 102 patients undergoing cyberknife fiducial free spinal radiosurgery. Outcomes measured included pain relief and complication rates. Treatment reduced median visual analog scale scores from 7 to 1 ($P<.001$). An overall complication incidence of 2% was reported, which mainly included incidences of segmental neuropathy due to tumor hemorrhage, and vertebral instability. Gerszten and colleagues[46] published a prospective case series (Class II evidence) of 500 patients who underwent radiosurgery for the treatment of spinal neoplasms. Parameters measured were functional outcome, pain relief, and tumor control. Eighty-five percent of patients with neurologic deficits before treatment exhibited improvement after treatment. An overall 86% of patients (which included both radiosensitive and radioresistant neoplasms) reported pain relief. Tumor control (measured both clinically and on imaging) was achieved on 86% of patients overall. Gibbs and colleagues[47] prospectively analyzed outcomes (Class II evidence) in 74 patients with 102 spinal metastases treated with radiosurgery. The main parameters reported were functional improvement and complication rates. The study reported that an overall 84% of patients experienced a functional improvement, with only 2% of patients demonstrating deteriorating function. Complications occurred in only 3 patients (4%), all of which were myelopathies.

Acutely presenting symptoms of cervical epidural spinal cord compression by a neoplasm can be temporized by treatment with corticosteroids. The goal of corticosteroid administration is to decrease localized intramedullary edema. Optimal dosing is controversial, and there are few high-quality evidence-based studies comparing dosing regimens in the setting of metastatic spine disease. A Class I evidence study by Vecht and colleagues[48] and a Class II evidence study by Heimdal and colleagues[49] compared the relative efficacy of high-dose (96 mg intravenously) with low-dose (10 mg intravenously) dexamethasone in improving neurologic outcomes. The Class I study by Vecht and colleagues[48] found increased efficacy, in terms of neurologic outcomes, for the low-dose dexamethasone (25% vs 8% rate of neurologic improvement). The Class II Study by Heimdal and colleagues[49] found equal efficacy of neurologic outcome for both low-dose and high-dose cohorts, but found significantly higher rates of complications and side effects for the high-dose dexamethasone group. Hence, although there may not be a neurologic improvement benefit to giving low-dose versus high-dose steroids, evidence shows that low-dose steroids may have better outcomes based on their decreased incidence of complications.

Chemohormonal therapy may be used in the setting of sensitive tumors and is most often used as adjuvant therapy given that it cannot itself treat spinal instability. Breast, thyroid, and small cell lung carcinomas are generally sensitive to chemotherapy whereas gastrointestinal tract, squamous cell carcinoma of the lung, and renal cell carcinoma neoplasms are generally not.[4,50–56] Tumor pathology obtained from biopsy can predict the susceptibility of a neoplasm to hormonal modulation. For example, determination of breast adenocarcinoma estrogen receptor status determines whether estrogen receptor modulation can be used as an adjuvant therapy.[54,57–59] Furthermore, it is not uncommon for metastatic prostate lesions to present with hormone-insensitive tumors despite the original pathology demonstrating a hormone sensitive neoplasm. This event most often represents a phenomenon known as "hormonal escape" in which the primary hormone sensitive tumor was unsuccessfully managed via hormonal modulation, resulting in the selection of hormone-resistant clones.[52,60,61]

Although not a primary method of treatment, bisphosphonate use in the setting of metastatic cervical spine disease is advocated, due to the ability of bisphosphonates to reduce the incidence of skeletal-related events (SREs). Specifically, Class I evidence exists demonstrating the efficacy of clonodrate, pamidronate, and zoledronate in decreasing the incidence of total SREs.[62–68] However, evidence suggest that not all bisphosphonates have a similar efficacy n reducing the incidence of

SREs specific to the spine, such as spinal cord compression. Rosen and colleagues[66] conducted a randomized controlled trial (Class I evidence) directly comparing the efficacy of zoledronate to pamidronate. The study found that zoledronate was more efficacious in reducing the incidence of both pathologic vertebral fractures and cord compression.

Indications for Surgery in Metastatic Cervical Tumors

The general indications for surgical intervention are (1) neurologic dysfunction, (2) spinal instability, and (3) intractable pain. Indication for surgical intervention in the upper cervical spine is most often attributable to spinal instability. As discussed previously, neurologic dysfunction in the setting of an upper cervical tumor is more indicative of cord compression from spinal instability rather than direct tumor cord compression. An occipitocervical fixation alone is most often sufficient, given that the compression is not due to direct tumor impingement, thereby not requiring a decompressive laminectomy. Surgery is indicated more often in the lower cervical spine than in the upper cervical spine, due to metastatic lesions localizing more often to the subaxial spine, the relatively narrower subaxial canal resulting in an earlier onset of neurologic deficit versus the upper cervical spine, and a greater subaxial segmental mobility resulting in increased risk of spinal instability.[16,69]

Although the staging scoring systems already discussed assist in indicating whether a palliative or curative surgery is most appropriate, palliative surgery is generally indicated in the setting of metastatic tumors. Curative surgery is mostly limited to primary spine tumors, but is possible in the rare cases of exceptionally isolated metastatic tumors. For example, the main indication for a curative wide surgical resection in the upper cervical spine is for treating predominantly isolated tumor to the posterior arch of C1 or C2. Nonetheless, even in such cases root and vertebral artery involvement must be considered, as it limits the aggressiveness of the surgical approach. In the case of root involvement, patients must be extensively informed about possible postoperative neurologic deficits in the upper limb if the root cannot be spared. The obstacle posed by the vertebral arteries can be managed by performing a unilateral or bilateral vascular bypass. Taking this approach underscores the necessity of obtaining a vertebral artery arteriography during the preoperative planning period.[16,69]

SURGICAL TECHNIQUES
Intralesional Vertebrectomy and Fixation

Truly the workhorse technique of cervical metastatic lesions, the anterior cervical corpectomy is a well-known approach to spine surgeons. Although it is beyond the scope of this review to discuss the specific details of this technique, there are several important caveats in the setting of metastatic lesions. First, in the setting of untreated lesions, the planes of dissection are often as would be expected with a standard anterior cervical approach. However, if the patient has been irradiated before surgery, it is suggested to potentially involve a head and neck surgeon to aid in the approach. Esophageal injury and swallowing dysfunction can lead to significant postoperative morbidity in any anterior cervical operation, but radiation-related scarring can significantly increase the risks of such complications. Second, in the setting of known highly vascularized lesions such as metastatic renal cell carcinoma, hepatocellular carcinoma, or thyroid carcinoma, vascular studies may be indicated prior to surgery. An angiogram may reveal large arterial feeding vessels from the vertebral arteries or, less commonly, the carotid arteries. Preoperative embolization may thus help avoid significant intraoperative hemorrhage. Finally, lesions may often involve multiple vertebral levels, and thus surgeons should be prepared to conduct multiple-level corpectomies if lytic lesions are extensive. In these cases it is suggested to supplement the anterior reconstruction with posterior stabilization as well.

Laminectomy and Fixation

This technique is less often used as the primary stand-alone technique, as most lesions of the subaxial spine are located anteriorly, which is generally easily approached. Therefore, this technique is usually supplementary following an anterior decompression and reconstruction. Given the poor quality of bone in cancer patients (cachexia, prior irradiation, and so forth), the likelihood of failure of the anterior instrumentation is increased in such patients. However, at the craniocervical junction, posterior decompression and stabilization is often the primary modality, as spinal compression in this area is more often associated with subluxation than with mass effect. Preoperative angiography is often very helpful in this area in delineating vertebral artery anatomy so as to avoid intraoperative tumor bleeding, to avoid inadvertent vertebral artery injury due to obliteration of normal anatomy by tumor involvement, and to prepare for potential vascular bypass if required to avoid perioperative stroke.

Partial or En Bloc Vertebrectomy

Vertebrectomy with negative margins, so-called en bloc vertebrectomy, is very rarely indicated in the cervical spine for metastatic lesions. In the setting of primary tumors, such as chordoma or sarcoma, en bloc resections pose substantial risks including neurologic dysfunction and vascular injury. Therefore, given that most metastatic lesions are approached with the goal of palliation, en bloc resections are generally not recommended in this area even if deemed feasible.

OUTCOMES FOR THE SURGICAL MANAGEMENT OF METASTATIC CERVICAL SPINE TUMORS

High-class evidence studies (Class I and Class II) addressing surgical outcomes are lacking in the literature. To date, the authors have identified only one Class I (randomized controlled trial) study[45] and two Class II prospective case studies[70,71] that include patients with cervical metastatic lesions reported in the literature. Of importance is that only one of the studies was exclusive in reporting outcomes for patients with metastatic cervical lesions.[71] Ten additional Class IV evidence retrospective studies[15,72–80] addressing surgical outcomes in managing metastatic cervical spine tumors are reported in the literature (**Table 2**).

The Class I evidence was conducted by Patchell and colleagues.[45] The study was a 10-year multi-institutional, nonblinded, randomized controlled trial to assess the efficacy of direct decompressive surgery for the treatment of spinal cord compression caused by metastatic cancer. The study enrolled a total of 123 patients, and ultimately 101 patients were evaluated. The 101 patients were randomized into two groups. The first group (n = 50, 5 afflicted with cervical lesions) was treated with surgery followed by radiotherapy. The second group (n = 51, 8 afflicted with cervical lesions) was treated with radiotherapy alone. The surgical approach used varied. Radiotherapy for both treatment groups was delivered in 10 3-Gy fractions, for a total of 30 Gy. The study found that significantly more patients in the surgery plus radiotherapy group (S) were able to ambulate in comparison to the radiotherapy group (R) alone after treatment (S: 84% vs R: 57%, $P = .001$). The study also found statistically higher rates of retention of ambulation, reacquisition of ambulation, American Spinal Injury Association muscle strength scores, and Frankel scores in the group treated with surgery and radiotherapy. The investigators also reported a significant difference in survival when comparing the radiotherapy-alone group with the surgery and radiotherapy group (S: 126 days median survival vs R: 100 days median survival; $P = .033$).[45] Pain alleviation outcomes, measured as mean daily morphine equivalents, were also superior in the surgery and radiotherapy group (S: $P = .002$). Although outcomes were supportive of surgical management in general, it must be noted that reported outcomes were not stratified to the cervical spine.

Class II evidence is reported by two studies. Ibrahim and colleagues[70] conducted a multicenter prospective study evaluating surgical efficacy in improving quality of life in patients with spinal metastases. The study enrolled 223 patients, 16% of whom were afflicted with cervical lesions. Neurologic outcomes measured included postoperative ambulation (98%) and the percentage of patients who regained ambulation postoperatively (55%). Of note, Ibrahim and colleagues[70] stratified neurologic outcomes according to the type of surgery undergone by patients (en bloc or debulking excision vs palliative surgery), and found that neurologic outcomes were best for patients undergoing excisional surgical management.

The Class II study by Quan and colleagues[71] was the only prospective study identified that specifically addressed outcomes of surgical management in patients with metastatic cervical spine lesions. The investigators reported the clinical outcomes of 26 consecutive patients undergoing surgery for symptomatic metastases of the cervical and cervicothoracic spine. All patients were followed up postoperatively at 1, 3, 6, and 12 months. Patients underwent palliative decompression and stabilization via anterior, posterior, or combined approach, depending on the topography of the lesion. The study found a statistically significant improvement in pain control and global health as scored by the EORTC QLQ-C30 questionnaire.[81] Of importance is that the study also noted that neurologic function was maintained, concluding that surgical intervention was an amenable method of preventing further neurologic decline. Outcomes reported by the identified retrospective Class IV studies are summarized in **Table 2**.

Based on available evidence, resection of cervical metastases with reconstruction and instrumented stabilization is an efficacious means for improving patient quality of life via decreased pain and improvement/preservation of physical functioning.

MANAGING COMPLICATIONS
Cerebrospinal Fluid Leak

Although CSF leaks are a potential risk in any cervical operation, the potential is increased with

Table 2
Summary of studies reporting retrospective outcomes in the surgical management of metastatic cervical spine disease

Study	Patient Size	Results		Mean Survival (mo)
Denaro et al,[15] 2011	46	Neurologic status	5/18 regained ambulation; 19/46 regained normal function (Frankel grade E); 1/46 worsened neurologically	27
Omeis et al,[80] 2010	5	Neurologic status	ASIA grade improved from 83.4 to 90.8	Not reported
		Pain	Mean VAS score reduced from 6.4 to 1	
Chuang et al,[74] 2008	17	Neurologic status	Mean increase in JOA scale: 3.1; mean improvement in Nurick scale: −0.31	10.6
		Pain	Mean improvement in Mankoski pain scale: 4.7	
Oda et al,[79] 2006	32	Neurological status	24/34 improved in Frankel grade; 16/18 regained ambulation	12.2
		Pain	32/32 experienced pain relief	
Liu et al,[77] 2005	6	Neurologic status	1/6 improved in neurologic deficit	Not reported
		Pain	5/6 experienced pain relief	
Heidecke et al,[75] 2003	62	Neurologic status	20/62 improved in Frankel grade; 4/62 decreased in Frankel grade	15
Miller et al,[83] 2000	29	Neurologic status	4/14 had complete resolution of gait impairment; 8/14 had improvement in gait impairment; 10/29 improved in Frankel grade	9.5
		Pain	15/25 had complete pain relief; 23/25 experienced some improvement in pain	
Caspar et al,[73] 1999	30	Neurologic status	19/19 had improvement in brachialgia; 16/16 had improvement in radiculopathy; 9/9 had improvement of myelopathy	35.8
		Pain	16/26 had complete relief of pain; 25/26 had improvement in pain	
Jonsson et al,[76] 1994	51	Neurologic status	5/6 had improvement in quadriparesis; 15/21 experienced complete resolution of radiculopathy; 21/21 had improvement in radiculopathy	12
Atanasiu et al,[72] 1993	20	Neurologic status	9/14 experienced improved neurologic deficit; 1/14 had worsening neurologic deficit	11
		Pain	11/20 had complete relief of pain; 19/20 experienced some relief of pain	

Abbreviations: ASIA, American Spinal Injury Association; JOA, Japanese Orthopedic Association; VAS, visual analog scale.

spinal tumor resections. First, prior irradiation can make the plane between the tumor and the dura exceptionally challenging. Second, extensive drilling may be required for decompression, which can put the dura at increased risk. Finally, dural repair can be challenging when tumor invades the dura. In such cases, postoperative CSF leaks can be persistent. In cases of prior irradiation or presumed dura invasion, patients should be prepared for prolonged lumbar drainage. In most

---

Box 1
Diagnosis and Management Pearls

Physicians treating cancer survivors with new progressive or severe mechanical neck pain should have a high suspicion for a new cervical metastatic lesion in such patients

Preoperative angiography should be considered in any metastatic lesion of the cervical spine to avoid intraoperative bleeding and prepare for potential bypass or ligation/embolizations procedures if thought to be beneficial

Anterior cervical corpectomy and fixation is the workhorse technique for most subaxial spine lesions, whereas laminectomy and posterior fixation is the primary technique for occipital-cervical and atlantoaxial lesions

Head and neck surgeons should be considered in obtaining anterior cervical access for patients with prior neck irradiation

Stereotactic radiation is now an option for recurrent or radioresistant tumors

---

cases, placement of an intraoperative lumbar drain is recommended so as to allow dural decompression with the initial direct dural repair.

Vertebral Artery Injury

Vertebral arterial bleeding intraoperatively can generally be controlled with pressure and ligation/clipping. Aneurysm clips or general vascular clips should be easily accessible for all cases of cervical spine tumors. However, unplanned ligation of such vessels to control bleeding can place patients at risk for perioperative stroke. If there is any concern preoperatively that the vertebral artery is significantly at risk, a formal angiogram should be done. This technique can help identify collateral circulation if a vessel needs to be sacrificed. In addition, if there are significant arterial feeders to the tumor, they can be embolized before surgery.

Esophageal Injury

Esophageal injury is a known risk with anterior cervical surgery that can lead to severe postoperative morbidity and potential mortality. In those patients with preoperative irradiation, esophageal tears can be more easily encountered. In these cases the authors usually ask for a head and neck surgeon to assist with the exposure. He or she can assist in dissecting the esophagus from the spine and can also provide a direct repair if problems are encountered.

SUMMARY

Metastatic cervical spine disease is not of rare occurrence, and providers managing cancer survivors should be suspicious of metastatic cervical lesions in such patients presenting with newly progressive or severe mechanical and/or nonmechanical pain (**Box 1**). The approach to a diagnosis should include a careful physical examination as well as a workup including plain radiographs, MRI, CT, and bone scintigraphy. Management is multidisciplinary and can be either nonoperative or operative. Ultimately, optimal management is dependent on appropriate patient selection for each of the available treatment modalities.

REFERENCES

1. Marchesi DG, Boos N, Aebi M. Surgical treatment of tumors of the cervical spine and first two thoracic vertebrae. J Spinal Disord 1993;6(6):489–96.
2. Fehlings MG, David KS, Vialle L, et al. Decision making in the surgical treatment of cervical spine metastases. Spine (Phila Pa 1976) 2009;34(Suppl 22): S108–17.
3. Cancer facts and figures 2005. Atlanta: American Cancer Society; 2005.
4. Sciubba DM, Petteys RJ, Dekutoski MB, et al. Diagnosis and management of metastatic spine disease. J Neurosurg Spine 2010;13(1):94–108.
5. Molina CA, Gokaslan ZL, Sciubba DM. Spinal tumors. In: Norden AD, Reardon DA, Wen PC, editors. Primary Central Nervous System Tumors. Humana Press; 2011. p. 529.
6. Cloyd JM, Chou D, Deviren V, et al. En bloc resection of primary tumors of the cervical spine: report of two cases and systematic review of the literature. Spine J 2009;9(11):928–35.
7. Chaichana KL, Pendleton C, Sciubba DM, et al. Outcome following decompressive surgery for different histological types of metastatic tumors causing epidural spinal cord compression. Clinical article. J Neurosurg Spine 2009;11(1):56–63.
8. Chaichana KL, Pendleton C, Wolinsky JP, et al. Vertebral compression fractures in patients presenting with metastatic epidural spinal cord compression. Neurosurgery 2009;65(2):267, 274 [discussion: 274–5].
9. Cybulski GR. Methods of surgical stabilization for metastatic disease of the spine. Neurosurgery 1989; 25(2):240–52.

10. York JE, Wildrick DM, Gokaslan ZL. Metastatic tumors. In: Benzel EC, Stillerman CB, editors. The Thoracic Spine. St Louis: Quality Medical Publishing; 1999. p. 392–411.

11. Jenis LG, Dunn EJ, An HS. Metastatic disease of the cervical spine. A review. Clin Orthop Relat Res 1999;(359):89–103.

12. Moulding HD, Bilsky MH. Metastases to the craniovertebral junction. Neurosurgery 2010;66(Suppl 3): 113–8.

13. Arguello F, Baggs RB, Duerst RE, et al. Pathogenesis of vertebral metastasis and epidural spinal cord compression. Cancer 1990;65(1):98–106.

14. Rao S, Badani K, Schildhauer T, et al. Metastatic malignancy of the cervical spine. A nonoperative history. Spine (Phila Pa 1976) 1992;17(Suppl 10):S407–12.

15. Denaro V, Di Martino A, Papalia R, et al. Patients with cervical metastasis and neoplastic pachymeningitis are less likely to improve neurologically after surgery. Clin Orthop Relat Res 2011;469(3):708–14.

16. Mazel C, Balabaud L, Bennis S, et al. Cervical and thoracic spine tumor management: surgical indications, techniques, and outcomes. Orthop Clin North Am 2009;40(1):75, 92, vi–vii.

17. Sundaresan N, Krol G, DiGiacinto G. Metastatic tumors of the spine. In: Sundaresan N, Schmidek H, Schiller A, editors. Tumors of the Spine. Diagnosis and Clinical Management. Philadelphia: WB Saunders; 1990.

18. Sundaresan N, Boriani S, Rothman A, et al. Tumors of the osseous spine. J Neurooncol 2004;69(1–3): 273–90.

19. Sherk HH. Lesions of the atlas and axis. Clin Orthop Relat Res 1975;(109):33–41.

20. George B, Lot G, Velut S, et al. French Language Society of Neurosurgery. 44th Annual Congress. Brussels, 8-12 June 1993. Tumors of the foramen magnum. Neurochirurgie 1993;39(Suppl 1):1–89.

21. Phillips E, Levine AM. Metastatic lesions of the upper cervical spine. Spine (Phila Pa 1976) 1989; 14(10):1071–7.

22. Ono K, Tada K. Metal prosthesis of the cervical vertebra. J Neurosurg 1975;42(5):562–6.

23. Sciubba DM, Gokaslan ZL. Diagnosis and management of metastatic spine disease. Surg Oncol 2006; 15(3):141–51.

24. Dickman CA, Spetzler RF, Sonntag VK. Surgery of the craniovertebral junction. New York: Thieme; 1998.

25. An HS, Vaccaro AR, Dolinskas CA, et al. Differentiation between spinal tumors and infections with magnetic resonance imaging. Spine (Phila Pa 1976) 1991;16(Suppl 8):S334–8.

26. Tomita T, Galicich JH, Sundaresan N. Radiation therapy for spinal epidural metastases with complete block. Acta Radiol Oncol 1983;22(2):135–43.

27. Donthineni R. Diagnosis and staging of spine tumors. Orthop Clin North Am 2009;40(1):1, 7, v.

28. Sciubba DM, Gallia GL, McGirt MJ, et al. Thoracic kyphotic deformity reduction with a distractible titanium cage via an entirely posterior approach. Neurosurgery 2007;60(4):223, 230 [discussion: 230–1].

29. Tokuhashi Y, Matsuzaki H, Toriyama S, et al. Scoring system for the preoperative evaluation of metastatic spine tumor prognosis. Spine 1990;15(11):1110–3.

30. Harrington KD. The use of methylmethacrylate for vertebral-body replacement and anterior stabilization of pathological fracture-dislocations of the spine due to metastatic malignant disease. J Bone Joint Surg Am 1981;63(1):36–46.

31. Kostuik J, Weinstein J. Differential diagnosis and surgical treatment of metastatic spine tumors. In: Frymoyer J, editor. The Adult Spine: Principles and Practice. New York: Raven Press; 1991. p. 861–88.

32. DeWald RL, Bridwell KH, Prodromas C, et al. Reconstructive spinal surgery as palliation for metastatic malignancies of the spine. Spine (Phila Pa 1976) 1985;10(1):21–6.

33. Boriani S, Weinstein J. Differential diagnosis and surgical treatment of primary benign and malignant neoplasms. In: Frymoyer J, editor. The adult spine: principles and practice. Philadelphia: Lippincott-Raven; 1997. p. 951–87.

34. Tomita K, Kawahara N, Baba H, et al. Total en bloc spondylectomy. A new surgical technique for primary malignant vertebral tumors. Spine (Phila Pa 1976) 1997;22(3):324–33.

35. Tokuhashi Y, Matsuzaki H, Oda H, et al. A revised scoring system for preoperative evaluation of metastatic spine tumor prognosis. Spine (Phila Pa 1976) 2005;30(19):2186–91.

36. Rades D, Huttenlocher S, Dunst J, et al. Matched pair analysis comparing surgery followed by radiotherapy and radiotherapy alone for metastatic spinal cord compression. J Clin Oncol 2010;28(22): 3597–604.

37. Kijima T, Fujii Y, Suyama T, et al. Radiotherapy to bone metastases from renal cell carcinoma with or without zoledronate. BJU Int 2009;103(5):620–4.

38. Niang U, Kamer S, Ozsaran Z, et al. The management of painful bone metastases with bisphosphonates and palliative radiotherapy: a retrospective evaluation of 372 cases. J BUON 2009;14(2): 245–9.

39. Rades D, Lange M, Veninga T, et al. Preliminary results of spinal cord compression recurrence evaluation (score-1) study comparing short-course versus long-course radiotherapy for local control of malignant epidural spinal cord compression. Int J Radiat Oncol Biol Phys 2009;73(1):228–34.

40. Rose PS, Laufer I, Boland PJ, et al. Risk of fracture after single fraction image-guided intensity-modulated radiation therapy to spinal metastases. J Clin Oncol 2009;27(30):5075–9.

41. Wowra B, Muacevic A, Zausinger S, et al. Radiosurgery for spinal malignant tumors. Dtsch Arztebl Int 2009;106(7):106–12.

42. Kaasa S, Brenne E, Lund JA, et al. Prospective randomised multicenter trial on single fraction radiotherapy (8 Gy × 1) versus multiple fractions (3 Gy × 10) in the treatment of painful bone metastases. Radiother Oncol 2006;79(3):278–84.

43. Nielsen OS, Bentzen SM, Sandberg E, et al. Randomized trial of single dose versus fractionated palliative radiotherapy of bone metastases. Radiother Oncol 1998;47(3):233–40.

44. Maranzano E, Bellavita R, Rossi R, et al. Short-course versus split-course radiotherapy in metastatic spinal cord compression: results of a phase III, randomized, multicenter trial. J Clin Oncol 2005;23(15):3358–65.

45. Patchell RA, Tibbs PA, Regine WF, et al. Direct decompressive surgical resection in the treatment of spinal cord compression caused by metastatic cancer: a randomised trial. Lancet 2005;366(9486):643–8.

46. Gerszten PC, Burton SA, Ozhasoglu C, et al. Radiosurgery for spinal metastases: clinical experience in 500 cases from a single institution. Spine (Phila Pa 1976) 2007;32(2):193–9.

47. Gibbs IC, Kamnerdsupaphon P, Ryu MR, et al. Image-guided robotic radiosurgery for spinal metastases. Radiother Oncol 2007;82(2):185–90.

48. Vecht CJ, Haaxma-Reiche H, van Putten WL, et al. Initial bolus of conventional versus high-dose dexamethasone in metastatic spinal cord compression. Neurology 1989;39(9):1255–7.

49. Heimdal K, Hirschberg H, Slettebo H, et al. High incidence of serious side effects of high-dose dexamethasone treatment in patients with epidural spinal cord compression. J Neurooncol 1992;12(2):141–4.

50. Harel R, Angelov L. Spine metastases: current treatments and future directions. Eur J Cancer 2010;46(15):2696–707.

51. Amato RJ, Hernandez-McClain J, Henary H. Bone-targeted therapy: phase II study of strontium-89 in combination with alternating weekly chemohormonal therapies for patients with advanced androgen-independent prostate cancer. Am J Clin Oncol 2008;31(6):532–8.

52. Kattan JG, Farhat FS, Chahine GY, et al. Weekly docetaxel, zoledronic acid and estramustine in hormone-refractory prostate cancer (HRPC). Invest New Drugs 2008;26(1):75–9.

53. Lin AM, Rini BI, Derynck MK, et al. A phase I trial of docetaxel/estramustine/imatinib in patients with hormone-refractory prostate cancer. Clin Genitourin Cancer 2007;5(5):323–8.

54. Cazzaniga ME, Dogliotti L, Cascinu S, et al. Diagnosis, management and clinical outcome of bone metastases in breast cancer patients: results from a prospective, multicenter study. Oncology 2006;71(5–6):374–81.

55. Beer TM, Garzotto M, Henner WD, et al. Intermittent chemotherapy in metastatic androgen-independent prostate cancer. Br J Cancer 2003;89(6):968–70.

56. Daliani DD, Assikis V, Tu SM, et al. Phase II trial of cyclophosphamide, vincristine, and dexamethasone in the treatment of androgen-independent prostate carcinoma. Cancer 2003;97(3):561–7.

57. Amir E, Ooi WS, Simmons C, et al. Discordance between receptor status in primary and metastatic breast cancer: an exploratory study of bone and bone marrow biopsies. Clin Oncol (R Coll Radiol) 2008;20(10):763–8.

58. Lipton A, Steger GG, Figueroa J, et al. Extended efficacy and safety of denosumab in breast cancer patients with bone metastases not receiving prior bisphosphonate therapy. Clin Cancer Res 2008;14(20):6690–6.

59. Paridaens RJ, Dirix LY, Beex LV, et al. Phase III study comparing exemestane with tamoxifen as first-line hormonal treatment of metastatic breast cancer in postmenopausal women: the European Organisation for Research and Treatment of Cancer Breast Cancer Cooperative Group. J Clin Oncol 2008;26(30):4883–90.

60. Nagata M, Ueda T, Komiya A, et al. Treatment and prognosis of patients with paraplegia or quadriplegia because of metastatic spinal cord compression in prostate cancer. Prostate Cancer Prostatic Dis 2003;6(2):169–73.

61. Zafeirakis A, Papatheodorou G, Arhontakis A, et al. Predictive implications of bone turnover markers after palliative treatment with (186)Re-HEDP in hormone-refractory prostate cancer patients with painful osseous metastases. Eur J Nucl Med Mol Imaging 2010;37(1):103–13.

62. Paterson AH, Powles TJ, Kanis JA, et al. Double-blind controlled trial of oral clodronate in patients with bone metastases from breast cancer. J Clin Oncol 1993;11(1):59–65.

63. Kristensen B, Ejlertsen B, Mouridsen HT, et al. Bisphosphonate treatment in primary breast cancer: results from a randomised comparison of oral pamidronate versus no pamidronate in patients with primary breast cancer. Acta Oncol 2008;47(4):740–6.

64. Hortobagyi GN, Theriault RL, Porter L, et al. Efficacy of pamidronate in reducing skeletal complications in patients with breast cancer and lytic bone metastases. Protocol 19 Aredia Breast Cancer Study Group. N Engl J Med 1996;335(24):1785–91.

65. Lipton A, Theriault RL, Hortobagyi GN, et al. Pamidronate prevents skeletal complications and is effective palliative treatment in women with breast carcinoma and osteolytic bone metastases: long term follow-up of two randomized, placebo-controlled trials. Cancer 2000;88(5):1082–90.

66. Rosen LS, Gordon D, Kaminski M, et al. Long-term efficacy and safety of zoledronic acid compared with pamidronate disodium in the treatment of skeletal complications in patients with advanced multiple myeloma or breast carcinoma: a randomized, double-blind, multicenter, comparative trial. Cancer 2003;98(8):1735–44.

67. Rosen LS, Gordon D, Tchekmedyian S, et al. Zoledronic acid versus placebo in the treatment of skeletal metastases in patients with lung cancer and other solid tumors: a phase III, double-blind, randomized trial–the Zoledronic Acid Lung Cancer and Other Solid Tumors Study Group. J Clin Oncol 2003;21(16):3150–7.

68. Saad F, Gleason DM, Murray R, et al. Long-term efficacy of zoledronic acid for the prevention of skeletal complications in patients with metastatic hormone-refractory prostate cancer. J Natl Cancer Inst 2004;96(11):879–82.

69. Hoshino Y, Kurokawa T, Nakamura K, et al. A report on the safety of unilateral vertebral artery ligation during cervical spine surgery. Spine (Phila Pa 1976) 1996;21(12):1454–7.

70. Ibrahim A, Crockard A, Antonietti P, et al. Does spinal surgery improve the quality of life for those with extradural (spinal) osseous metastases? An international multicenter prospective observational study of 223 patients. J Neurosurg Spine 2008;8(3):271–8.

71. Quan GM, Vital JM, Pointillart V. Outcomes of palliative surgery in metastatic disease of the cervical and cervicothoracic spine. J Neurosurg Spine 2011; 14(5):612–8.

72. Atanasiu JP, Badatcheff F, Pidhorz L. Metastatic lesions of the cervical spine. A retrospective analysis of 20 cases. Spine (Phila Pa 1976) 1993;18(10):1279–84.

73. Caspar W, Pitzen T, Papavero L, et al. Anterior cervical plating for the treatment of neoplasms in the cervical vertebrae. J Neurosurg 1999;90(Suppl 1):27–34.

74. Chuang HC, Wei ST, Lee HC, et al. Preliminary experience of titanium mesh cages for pathological fracture of middle and lower cervical vertebrae. J Clin Neurosci 2008;15(11):1210–5.

75. Heidecke V, Rainov NG, Burkert W. Results and outcome of neurosurgical treatment for extradural metastases in the cervical spine. Acta Neurochir (Wien) 2003;145(10):873, 880. [discussion: 880–1].

76. Jonsson B, Jonsson H Jr, Karlstrom G, et al. Surgery of cervical spine metastases: a retrospective study. Eur Spine J 1994;3(2):76–83.

77. Liu JK, Rosenberg WS, Schmidt MH. Titanium cage-assisted polymethylmethacrylate reconstruction for cervical spinal metastasis: technical note. Neurosurgery 2005;56(Suppl 1):E207 [discussion: E207].

78. Mazel C, Hoffmann E, Antonietti P, et al. Posterior cervicothoracic instrumentation in spine tumors. Spine (Phila Pa 1976) 2004;29(11):1246–53.

79. Oda I, Abumi K, Ito M, et al. Palliative spinal reconstruction using cervical pedicle screws for metastatic lesions of the spine: a retrospective analysis of 32 cases. Spine (Phila Pa 1976) 2006;31(13): 1439–44.

80. Omeis I, Bekelis K, Gregory A, et al. The use of expandable cages in patients undergoing multilevel corpectomies for metastatic tumors in the cervical spine. Orthopedics 2010;33(2):87–92.

81. Aaronson NK, Ahmedzai S, Bergman B, et al. The European Organization for Research and Treatment of Cancer QLQ-C30: a quality-of-life instrument for use in international clinical trials in oncology. J Natl Cancer Inst 1993;85(5):365–76.

82. Hart RA, Boriani S, Biagini R, et al. A system for surgical staging and management of spine tumors. A clinical outcome study of giant cell tumors of the spine. Spine (Phila Pa 1976) 1997;22(15):1773, 1782 [discussion: 1783].

83. Miller DJ, Lang FF, Walsh GL, et al. Coaxial double-lumen methylmethacrylate reconstruction in the anterior cervical and upper thoracic spine after tumor resection. J Neurosurg 2000;92(Suppl 2): 181–90.

Management of Cervical Spine Trauma: Can a Prognostic Classification of Injury Determine Clinical Outcomes?

Melvin D. Helgeson, MD, David Gendelberg, BS,
Gursukhman S. Sidhu, MBBS, D. Greg Anderson, MD,
Alexander R. Vaccaro, MD, PhD*

KEYWORDS

- Subaxial injury classification • SLIC
- Discoligamentous complex • Neurologic injury
- Subaxial cervical spine

Cervical spine trauma remains one of the most common causes of morbidity in the United States with a significant financial burden on our society. For example, the estimated lifetime cost for a low tetraplegic injury (C5-C8) in a 25 year old will be more than $3 million.[1] Attempts to minimize the damage to the cervical spinal cord can result in very important improvements in the quality of life for these devastating injuries. Therefore, the goal of any surgeon is to appropriately identify those injuries that would benefit from surgical stabilization and decompression. Multiple classification systems have been developed by experts to assist others, and the purpose of any classification system is to provide insight into the injury pattern, severity, and prognosis. Unfortunately, traditional classification systems generally sought to describe the injury in great detail but overlooked the more important prognostic value of the neurologic status of patients. The Thoracolumbar Injury Classification System and subsequently the cervical spine with the Subaxial Injury Classification System (SLIC) have been developed to address the deficiencies of other classification schemes. With the introduction of these newer classification systems, the focus in spine trauma has moved to include injury pattern, severity, and neurologic status, thus, providing a better platform for clinicians to define treatment approaches and prognosis. The purpose of this article is to review the traditional and newer classification systems for the subaxial cervical spine and discuss the recent evidence to support the SLIC as a prognostic tool for spine surgeons.

TRADITIONAL CLASSIFICATION SYSTEMS

Sir Frank Holdsworth published the first detailed description of subaxial cervical spine trauma in 1970 based on his extensive experience in more than 1000 patients with quadriplegia/paraplegia and many more without spinal cord injury.[2] In his experience, specific fracture patterns were classified as either stable (simple wedge, burst, and extension injuries) or unstable (dislocations, rotational-fracture dislocations, and shear fractures), and patients were treated based on the injury morphology. During his vast experience, he

---

Department of Orthopaedic Surgery, Rothman Institute, Thomas Jefferson University and Hospitals, 925 Chestnut Street, Philadelphia, PA 19107, USA
* Corresponding author.
E-mail address: Alexvaccaro3@aol.com

Orthop Clin N Am 43 (2012) 89–96
doi:10.1016/j.ocl.2011.08.005
0030-5898/12/$ – see front matter © 2012 Elsevier Inc. All rights reserved.

also found that the posterior ligamentous complex was an important structure stabilizing the spine and used it to differentiate between the stable and unstable injuries. Although he dedicated a significant amount of energy into the management of neurologic injuries and how they relate to the patients' prognoses, he did not incorporate the neurologic status into his classification scheme. He undoubtedly managed patients based on their level of neurologic dysfunction but the classification system failed to reflect this, limiting the value of this scheme when generalized to the spine surgical community.

Allen and Ferguson[3] expanded the descriptive terms initiated by Holdsworth to include several other morphologic variables. In their classification system, the common fracture mechanisms were as follows: compression flexion, vertical compression, distractive flexion, compressive extension, distractive extension, and lateral flexion. They associated neurologic injury with the mechanism of injury and attempted to dictate a treatment plan based on the mechanism of injury. Although the mechanism of injury is associated with the neurologic injury, the mechanism was not predictive of final outcome and, therefore, not always useful in directing treatment. Harris and colleagues[4] modified this descriptive classification system to include the rotational vectors in 1986, but unfortunately the spotlight remained on injury morphology. Additionally, the mechanisms proposed were generally not validated biomechanically but were rather deduced on the bases of radiographic views. Some injuries fail to fit neatly into a specific category, perhaps because of complex or multidirectional force vectors that produced the spinal trauma.

The previous classifications systems focused on descriptive terminology and in doing so became cumbersome and less reliable. When evaluated by members of the Spine Trauma Study Group (STSG), there was only a 65% and 57% agreement among raters for the Ferguson/Allen and Harris classification systems, respectively.[5] The focus was firmly placed on injury morphology, with attempts to fit the fracture pattern into one of these previously determined categories. Frequently, fractures result from a mechanism that does not exactly correlate with one of the groups described by Harris, leaving ambiguity in the assessment of the injury.

SUBAXIAL INJURY CLASSIFICATION SYSTEM

In 2007, recognizing the difficulty with these traditional classification systems, the STSG sought to create a simple yet useful classification system for subaxial injuries in the cervical spine. The STSG recently derived a novel classification system for thoracolumbar injuries that was well received and easily adopted by the spine community.[6] They took the lessons learned from this previous classification system and incorporated them into the cervical spine, which created a paradigm shift in the thinking of cervical spine trauma. The focus was placed on neurologic injury and discoligamentous complex (DLC) in addition to the injury morphology. There are 6 variables that must be considered when describing a cervical spine injury:

1. Spinal level
2. Injury morphology (major category)
3. Bony injury description (ie, spinous process, lamina, lateral mass, superior facet, inferior facet, pedicle, transverse process, vertebral body)
4. Discoligamentous complex status (major category)
5. Neurologic status (major category)
6. Confounding variables (ie, diffused idiopathic hyperostosis, ankylosing spondylitis, osteoporosis, previous surgery, preexisting myelopathy/stenosis)

In this new classification system, the injury morphology, DLC, and neurologic injury are each evaluated separately and given a point value based on the level of severity (**Table 1**). Although each of these independent variables correlates with clinical outcome, the sum of the 3 values

Table 1
Subaxial Injury Classification System

Characteristic	Points
Injury morphology	
Compression	1
Burst	+1
Distraction	3
Translation/rotation	4
DLC	
Intact	0
Indeterminate	1
Disrupted	2
Neurologic status	
Intact	0
Root injury	1
Complete cord injury	2
Incomplete cord injury	3
Ongoing cord compression	+1

can be used to dictate care and determine prognosis.

Injury Morphology

Similar to previous classifications systems, the SLIC attempted to categorize the injury morphology but with a simplified approach to make it more useful. Using plain radiographs, computed tomography (CT), and magnetic resonance imaging (MRI), the fracture patterns were divided into 3 major categories in order of severity: compression, distraction, and translation/rotation.

Compressive injuries are judged as those with less vertebral height compared with the adjacent levels. Included in this category are simple compression fractures resulting in loss of height anteriorly and burst fractures. Burst fractures receive an additional point reflecting their increased instability compared with compression fractures. Flexion compression injuries or teardrop fractures are included in this category. Also included are minimally displaced lateral mass and facet fractures without any evidence of translation/rotation and they are likely the result of a lateral compression-type mechanism.

Distraction injuries are defined as any injury that results in distraction across the fracture, intervertebral disk, or posterior elements. These injuries are inherently unstable and are commonly seen with a distraction-extension–type mechanism. Although a CT scan can frequently determine if there is a distraction, an MRI can discover more subtle distraction injuries across the intervertebral disk. Also included in this category are any injuries that result in perched facets without frank dislocation or translation.

The final and most unstable injury pattern is rotation/translation, which is defined as abnormal translation of one vertebral body relative to the next. In their landmark work on cervical spine stability, White and Panjabi determined that any translation greater than 3.5 mm or angulation greater than 11° relative to the adjacent level is abnormal in the cervical spine.[7] The most common example of a rotation/translation injury is a dislocated facet. Also included in this category are bilateral pedicle fractures resulting in a traumatic spondylolisthesis or ipsilateral pedicle and lamina fractures resulting in a floating lateral mass and rotational deformity of one vertebrae relative to the adjacent vertebrae.

Compressive injuries are assigned 1 point, distraction injuries are assigned 3 points, and fracture/dislocations are assigned 4 points, with a burst fracture adding an additional point.

Discoligamentous Complex

Holdsworth previously discussed the importance of the posterior ligamentous complex but did not incorporate it into his classification system except to use the ligamentous status to determine stability.[2] The SLIC is the first classification system to place emphasis on the DLC by separating it as a distinct variable with an associated point value. The DLC can be graded as intact, indeterminate, or disrupted. The DLC is defined as the soft tissues supporting the articulation between 2 vertebra: the intervertebral disk, anterior longitudinal ligament, posterior longitudinal ligament, ligamentum flavum, interspinous ligament, supraspinous ligament, and the facet capsules. Any disruption of these structures results in instability between the 2 vertebra. Additionally, a ligamentous injury is less likely to heal compared with a bony injury and, therefore, more likely requires surgery to prevent long-term deformity.

In cases of facet dislocations, the facet capsules and the DLC are obviously disrupted but it is often more subtle. Abnormal facet alignment defined as less than 50% articular apposition or greater than 2 mm diastasis is associated with disruption of the DLC. Additionally, more subtle CT findings that may correlate with DLC disruption include disk space widening, interspinous widening, or vertebral rotation. With improvements in MRI technology, our ability to assess the DLC has improved dramatically, but there are still cases that are difficult to interpret with MRI and it should be judged as indeterminate.

An intact DLC is assigned 0 points, indeterminate is assigned 1 point, and disrupted is assigned 2 points.

Neurologic Injury

The final and possibly the most important predictor of clinical outcome is the presenting neurologic examination. Not only does the initial neurologic examination correlate directly with final outcome but it also correlates with spinal stability. In order for most patients to develop a neurologic deficit, a significant amount of force has to be transmitted through the spine and, in doing so, the supporting osteoligamentous structures become disrupted. This component is a key part of the SLIC, distinguishing it from all previous classification systems. Furthermore, patients with a neurologic deficit are more likely to require and undergo a decompressive procedure. The neurologic examination can be divided into the following categories in order of severity/urgency: intact, root injury, complete spinal cord injury, and incomplete spinal cord injury. Incomplete spinal cord injuries are rated as more severe because they require more emergent attention and are more likely to require a surgical procedure/decompression.

Zero points are assigned if the neurologic status is intact, whereas 1 point is assigned if there is a root injury, 2 points are assigned if there is a complete spinal cord injury, and 3 points are assigned if there is an incomplete spinal cord injury. An additional point is added if there is ongoing spinal cord compression.

CURRENT EVIDENCE TO SUPPORT THE SLIC

Although the SLIC has only been available for the past 4 years, there is already a significant amount of evidence to support its use as a prognostic tool. The first step with any classification system is to determine if it can be reliably used by an individual and between individuals. When initially publishing the classification system, the STSG compared it with the Harris and Ferguson/Allen systems and found that it compared favorably.[5] The interrater reliability for the SLIC was moderate (intraclass correlation [ICC] = 0.71) compared with moderate for both the Harris and Ferguson/Allen systems (κ = 0.41 and κ = 0.53, respectively). Furthermore, the intrarater reliability for the SLIC (ICC = 0.83) was better compared with the Harris and Ferguson/Allen systems (κ = 0.53 and κ = 0.63, respectively).

After proving the SLIC was reliable, the next step was to determine if it could adequately predict cases requiring surgical intervention. The same reviewers that determined the reliability of the SLIC were asked if a case was surgical or not and compared this answer with the numerical value assigned to the case using the SLIC. If the cases with a score of 5 or more were assumed to be operative and a score of 3 or less assumed to be nonoperative, there was a 93.3% agreement with the reviewers' opinion.[5] Therefore, the SLIC was predictive of the best course of treatment determined by experts in spine trauma 93% of the time.

Based on the prognostic ability of the SLIC, the STSG developed a detailed treatment algorithm for each type of injury, including compression/burst fractures, distraction injuries, translational/rotation injuries, and central cord syndrome.[8] According to the algorithm, the best approach for a compression/burst fracture would be an anterior approach. Compression or burst fractures typically score a 1 or a 2 combined for injury morphology and DLC status, and, therefore, the surgical decision is based on the neurologic status. Furthermore, if patients are neurologically intact, the total score would be less than 3 and

nonoperative treatment would be recommended; conversely, if there is ongoing compression (+1) and an incomplete spinal cord injury (3) associated with a burst fracture, the total score would be 6 and surgery would be recommended. As another example, an extension-distraction injury with disruption of the anterior longitudinal ligament/intervertebral disk would be assigned a value of 3 for injury morphology and 2 for DLC status. Therefore, surgery would be recommended regardless of the neurologic status. Finally, Dvorak and colleagues[8] concluded that the more severe cases of translation/rotation injuries are best treated posteriorly or with a combined anterior/posterior approach because of their severe instability. In another review by Patel and colleagues,[9] the SLIC was found to be the optimal classification system for subaxial trauma, and they illustrated this in several case examples.

In a recent study by Bono and colleagues,[10] they found that the intrarater reliability for the SLIC was 72.8% and the interrater reliability was 56.4%. Although their study also demonstrated the difficulty in determining exact fracture patterns, such as tear-drop fractures, the beauty of the SLIC is that this is not required. The injury morphology is simply graded as compressive, distraction, or translation/rotation.

SUMMARY

In creating the SLIC, the STSG has provided the spine community with a classification system with the versatility to apply across all subaxial cases, simple enough to actually be used, and effective at predicting clinical outcomes. Additional prospective studies would further substantiate these claims, but as of right now, it seems to be the best classification system available for subaxial cervical spine trauma.

TIPS/PEARLS

1. The 3 main contributors in determining surgical intervention are injury morphology, DLC status, and neurologic examination.
2. Neurologic status is a major predictor of clinical outcome.
3. If at all unsure about the status of the DLC on MRI, select indeterminate.
4. Simple fracture patterns, such as an isolated lateral mass fracture, are considered compressive injuries (likely resulting from lateral compression).
5. More complex fracture patterns, such as a floating lateral mass, can represent a rotational injury, and displacement from one

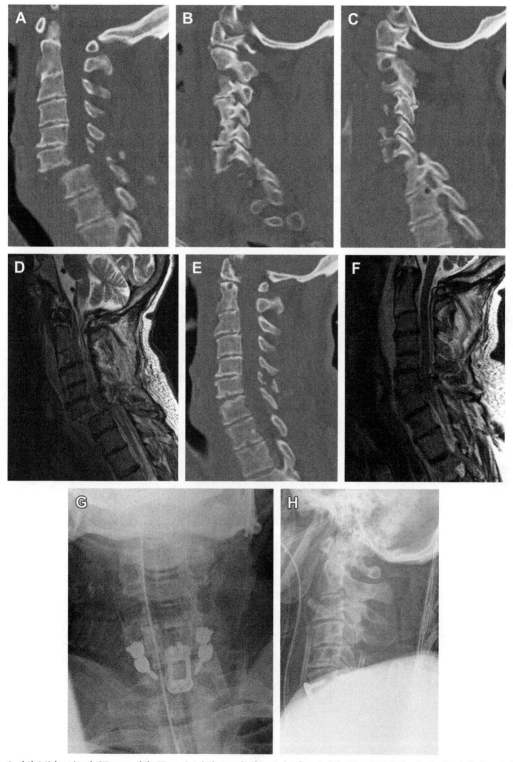

Fig. 1. (*A*) Midsagittal CT scan, (*B*) CT sagittal through the right facet, (*C*) CT sagittal through the left facet. (*D*) Sagittal T2 MRI revealed ongoing cord compression at C6–7. Following closed reduction, repeat CT scan (*E*) and MRI (*F*). (*G*, *H*) Postoperative anteroposterior (AP) and lateral radiographs.

vertebra to another should be carefully assessed.

CASE EXAMPLES
Case 1

An 85-year-old male driver involved in a head-on collision (with airbag deployment) presented at an outside hospital with initial loss of motor and sensory function in bilateral lower (BLE) and upper (BUE) extremities. Shortly after arrival, he began to regain function in his lower extremities and was transferred to our facility for definitive management. On arrival, his neurologic status revealed near full strength in BLE, but he continued to have weakness in BUE below the level of C6. Therefore, he was considered an incomplete

spinal cord injury. CT was immediately obtained revealing a bilateral facet dislocation at C6–7. **Fig. 1**A is a midsagittal CT scan, **Fig. 1**B is a CT sagittal through the right facet, and **Fig. 1**C is a CT sagittal through the left facet. **Fig. 1**D shows a sagittal T2 MRI that revealed ongoing cord compression at C6–7. Additionally, there is obvious disruption of the discoligamentous complex.

Therefore, on initial presentation to the authors' facility, this patient would have received an injury morphology score of 4, a DLC status score of 2, and a neurologic status score of 4, for a total SLIC score of 10, clearly supporting operative intervention. Following closed reduction, repeat CT scan (see **Fig. 1**E) and MRI (see **Fig. 1**F) did not reveal any further evidence of spinal cord

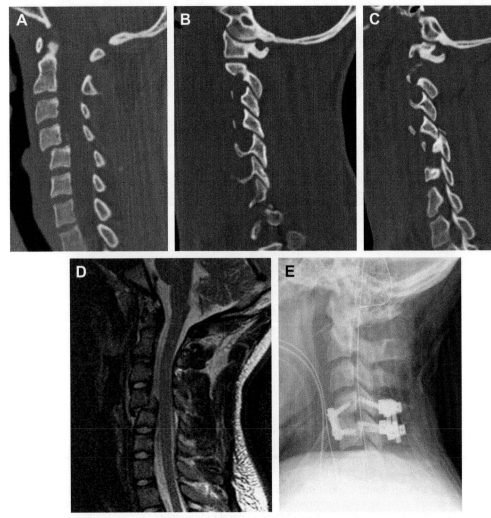

Fig. 2. (A) Midsagittal CT scan, (B) CT sagittal through the right facet, (C) CT sagittal through the left facet. There is a large disk fragment behind the vertebral body of C4 dictating an anterior surgical approach (D). (E) Postoperative lateral radiograph.

compression, reducing the SLIC score to 9 (neurologic examination unchanged) but still indicating surgical intervention is warranted.

Therefore, this patient underwent a posterior stabilization procedure (C6 lateral mass and C7 pedicle screws) followed by an anterior cervical discectomy and fusion. **Fig. 1**G and H show the postoperative anteroposterior (AP) and lateral radiographs.

On postoperative day 6, he was discharged to a rehabilitation facility. By the time of the discharge, he had near full strength except in the triceps and finger flexors bilaterally.

Case 2

A 15-year-old football player tackles another player with his head first (spear tackle) and presents with severe neck pain. He denies any numbness, tingling, weakness, or pain in BUE or BLE. A CT scan was obtained that demonstrates a unilateral facet dislocation. **Fig. 2**A shows a midsagittal CT scan, **Fig. 2**B shows a CT sagittal through the right facet, and **Fig. 2**C shows a CT sagittal through the left facet.

Sagittal MRI reveals no significant cord compression but obvious disruption of the DLC. Additionally, there is a large disk fragment behind the vertebral body of C4 dictating an anterior surgical approach (see **Fig. 2**D).

Therefore, this patient would receive an injury morphology score of 4 for translation/rotation, 2 for disruption of the DLC, and 0 for neurologic status, yielding a combined SLIC score of 6. Therefore, he underwent anterior cervical discectomy/decompression and fusion followed by posterior stabilization. **Fig. 2**E shows the postoperative lateral radiograph.

Case 3

A 16-year-old wrestler who landed on his head sustained the mild onset of neck pain. He continued to wrestle but had to stop because of persistent neck pain. He was diagnosed with a neck strain until plain radiographs were obtained 2 days later revealing interspinous widening across C4-5. An MRI was obtained revealing the evidence of distraction posteriorly and disruption of the posterior ligamentous structures. **Fig. 3**A, B

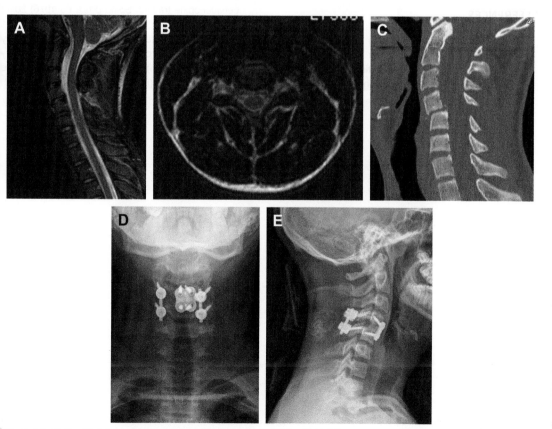

Fig. 3. (*A, B*) Sagittal MRI and axial MRI through C4-5. (*C*) Sagittal CT scan now revealing increased translation and angulation across C4-5. (*D, E*) Postoperative AP/lateral radiographs.

shows a sagittal MRI and an axial MRI through C4-5.

Given his normal neurologic examination, he received 3 points for distraction injury morphology and 2 points for the disruption of the DLC, giving a total SLIC score of 5. He was managed at an outside facility nonoperatively (SLIC score would have recommended surgical intervention) until repeat imaging was obtained 5 weeks later revealing the progression of his deformity and bilateral perched facets. **Fig.** 3C is the sagittal CT scan now revealing the increased translation and angulation across C4-5. The early evidence of fracture callous is also noted.

Given the progression of deformity, he was taken to the operating room for a C4-5 anterior cervical discectomy and fusion followed by a C4-5 posterior cervical fusion. Given that he was already showing evidence of fracture callous, the decision was made to start anteriorly and attempt reduction followed by a posterior stabilization procedure. As seen in the images, the authors were unable to obtain a complete reduction. **Fig.** 3D, E shows the postoperative AP and lateral radiographs.

REFERENCES

1. NSCIS. Spinal cord injury facts and figures at a glance. Birmingham (AL): Center NSCIS; 2011.
2. Holdsworth F. Fractures, dislocations, and fracture-dislocations of the spine. J Bone Joint Surg Am 1970;52:1534.
3. Allen BL Jr, Ferguson RL, Lehmann TR, et al. A mechanistic classification of closed, indirect fractures and dislocations of the lower cervical spine. Spine (Philadelphia Pa 1976) 1982;7:1.
4. Harris JH Jr, Edeiken-Monroe B, Kopaniky DR. A practical classification of acute cervical spine injuries. Orthop Clin North Am 1986;17:15.
5. Vaccaro AR, Hulbert RJ, Patel AA, et al. The subaxial cervical spine injury classification system: a novel approach to recognize the importance of morphology, neurology, and integrity of the disco-ligamentous complex. Spine (Phila Pa 1976) 2007;32:2365.
6. Vaccaro AR, Lehman RA Jr, Hurlbert RJ, et al. A new classification of thoracolumbar injuries: the importance of injury morphology, the integrity of the posterior ligamentous complex, and neurologic status. Spine (Phila Pa 1976) 2005;30:2325.
7. White AA, Panjabi MM. Clinical biomechanics of the spine. 2nd edition. Philadelphia: Lippincott; 1990.
8. Dvorak MF, Fisher CG, Fehlings MG, et al. The surgical approach to subaxial cervical spine injuries: an evidence-based algorithm based on the SLIC classification system. Spine (Phila Pa 1976) 2007;32:2620.
9. Patel AA, Hurlbert RJ, Bono CM, et al. Classification and surgical decision making in acute subaxial cervical spine trauma. Spine (Phila Pa 1976) 2010;35:S228.
10. Bono CM, Schoenfeld A, Gupta G, et al. Reliability and reproducibility of SCIDS (subaxial cervical injury description system): a standardized nomenclature schema. Spine (Phila Pa 1976) 2011;36(17):E1140–4.

Cervical Total Disk Replacement: Complications and Avoidance

Behnam Salari, DO, MS[a,b], Paul C. McAfee, MD, MBA[a,b],*

KEYWORDS

- Cervical total disk replacement • Complications
- Indications

Anterior cervical diskectomy and fusion (ACDF) for patients with neurologic deficits, radicular arm pain, and neck pain refractory to conservative management are successful.[1] The approach and procedure were first described by Robinson and Smith in 1955[2] and have become the anterior cervical standard of care for orthopedic surgeons and neurosurgeons. This has led to advancements and innovations to address disease processes of the cervical spine with motion-preserving technology. The possibility of obtaining the goals of an anterior cervical decompression while maintaining adjacent segment motion led to the advent of cervical total disk replacement (TDR). Currently the Food and Drug Administration (FDA) has approved 3 cervical devices, Prestige (Medtronic Sofamor Danek, Memphis, TN, USA), Bryan (Medtronic Sofamor Danek), and ProDisc-C (Synthes, West Chester, PA, USA) with other investigational device exemption (IDE) trials under way (**Table 1**).

Adjacent level degenerative changes after ACDF may result from changes in the cervical spine biomechanics. Studies have reported that fusion causes increased biomechanical stresses at adjacent levels.[3–6] Symptomatic adjacent segment disease incidence has been reported as 2.9% per year, with new disease defined as the onset of radiculopathy or myelopathy requiring surgical management.[7] The levels most likely to develop adjacent segment disease were C5-C6 and C6-C7. Although significant, adjacent segment disease is not the only morbidity associated with cervical fusion. Concerns regarding graft donor site morbidity, decreased cervical range of motion, and pseudarthrosis have been recognized as well.[8–10] The reported theoretic advantages of cervical TDR will obviate the concerns and morbidities associated with anterior cervical fusion by preserving kinematics at the operative and adjacent levels without the need for fusion and bone graft. Although these theoretic benefits may be an advantage, approach-related complications are similar to those of anterior cervical fusion.

As TDR technology has progressed with an increased variety and evolution of cervical implants available, so has the progression of surgical techniques with identification and management of adverse events. Contraindications and indications for cervical TDR have been established.[11–15] These guidelines have been reported and recognized as possible causes of failure if not adhered to. Furthermore, complications and failure of cervical TDR can be related to both patient and surgeon factors. Implant failure arising from these factors can be identified, and with proper intraoperative technique, successful results can be achieved.

Disclosures: NuVasive Consultant, Globus Consultant (PCM).
a The Spine and Scoliosis Center, St. Joseph's Hospital, 7505 Osler Drive, Towson, MD 21204, USA
b Department of Orthopaedic Surgery, Orthopaedic Associates of Towson, O'Dea Medical Arts Building, Suite 104, 7505 Osler Drive, Towson, MD 21204, USA
* Corresponding author. Department of Orthopaedic Surgery, Orthopaedic Associates of Towson, O'Dea Medical Arts Building, Suite 104, 7505 Osler Drive, Towson, MD 21204.
E-mail address: mack8132@gmail.com

Orthop Clin N Am 43 (2012) 97–107
doi:10.1016/j.ocl.2011.08.006
0030-5898/12/$ – see front matter © 2012 Elsevier Inc. All rights reserved.

Table 1
Summary of cervical total disk replacement implants

Implant	Manufacturer
Bryan cervical disk[a]	Medtronic Sofamor Danek (Memphis, TN)
Prestige cervical disk[a]	Medtronic Sofamor Danek (Memphis, TN)
ProDisc-C[a]	Synthes Spine (West Chester, PA)
PCM cervical disk	NuVasive (San Diego, CA)
CerviCore disk	Stryker Spine (Allendale, NJ)
SECURE-C	Globus Medical (Audubon, PA)
DISCOVER disk	Depuy Spine (Raynham, MA)

[a] FDA approved.

TOTAL DISK REPLACEMENT RATIONALE

To focus on addressing the biomechanical issues that may arise from ACDF, cervical TDR has developed and undergone motion-preserving design changes that have included metal alloy and polyethylene-bearing surfaces. Design and function of TDR implants are directed in preserving motion at cervical disease segments, not restoration of motion in a degenerative segment (**Fig. 1**).

Concerns regarding adjacent segment disease arose from the concept that loss of motion at a fused segment leads to increased range of motion and intradiscal pressures at adjacent levels.[3,16] Goffin and colleagues[17] reported a 92% incidence of degeneration at adjacent levels after ACDF. Furthermore, Hillibrand and colleagues[7] reported a cumulative risk of 25% for adjacent segment disease at 10 years after ACDF. The pathology of these findings has been attributed to the natural progression of the disease process and postsurgical biomechanical changes at adjacent levels. Although the specific underlying cause of adjacent segment disease after fusion has not been identified, prevention with TDR is a possibility. Garrido and colleagues[18] presented a prospective randomized study of 46 patients enrolled in the Bryan TDR IDE study. Analysis of the arthrodesis group demonstrated significantly more ossification at the adjacent level than the Bryan TDR group 2 years postoperatively ($P = .003$) and 4-years postoperatively ($P = .004$). The study demonstrated that cervical TDR is associated with a lower incidence of adjacent level ossification than ACDF with plate fixation at both 2 years and 4 years postoperatively.

As discussed previously, TDR obviates harvesting autograft and the risk of viral transmission associated with allograft. Donor site morbidity from autograft harvesting for fusion has been a concern. Complications include donor site pain, infection, and pelvic fracture.[19–21] To

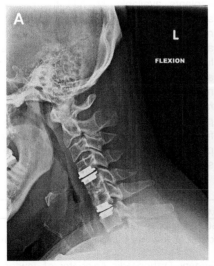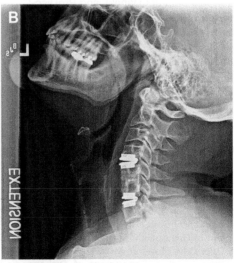

Fig. 1. (A) Flexion and (B) extension lateral radiographs of a 45-year-old man who underwent an ACDF previously. Unfortunately he developed adjacent segment disease with symptomatic cervical spondylosis at C4-C5 and C6-C7 by 2 years postoperatively. This was successfully treated with a ProDisc cervical disk arthroplasty above and below the ACDF level. Flexion and extension radiographs demonstrating motion at both cervical arthroplasty levels.

avoid these complications, premanufactured allograft supplements have been introduced as an alternative to autografts.[22] These come with the risk of disease transmission and must be addressed preoperatively with patients. Further concerns with allograft substitutes include higher rates of graft subsidence, nonunions, and delayed unions.[23–27] Together these factors influence yet another complication encountered with ACDF, pseudarthrosis. Rates of pseudarthrosis vary and are directly related to number of fusion levels. The clinical effects of pseudarthrosis on outcomes are correlated with loss of cervical alignment and foraminal distraction. Single-level ACDF pseudarthrosis rates range vary in the literature and are reported as high as 27% in multilevel surgery.[1]

With cervical TDR, the preserved motion innovation can avoid the complications and limitations of anterior cervical fusion. Direct decompression and removal of cervical pathologic disk can be accomplished as well as maintaining spinal kinematics. Theoretically this may prevent adjacent segment disease and additional operative intervention. Concurrently, cervical alignment, height, and decompression can be obtained with proper surgical technique. Further long-term clinical trials will establish the viability of this motion-preserving technology and its role as an alternative to spinal fusion.

SURGICAL APPROACH COMPLICATIONS

Despite the concerns identified with anterior cervical fusion, there is parallelism in approach-related complications with cervical TDR. The overall frequency and types of complications associated with the anterior approach for cervical arthroplasty will become more prevalent as investigational studies are completed. Intraoperative and postoperative approach-related events with anterior cervical spine surgery include esophageal injury, vertebral artery injury, vertebral body fracture, dysphagia/dysphonia, and dural tear. Immediate postoperative complications may result from airway compromise due to hematoma formation or edema. Complications from anterior spine surgery are not limited to the aforementioned events and with meticulous surgical technique and strategies these events can be recognized and controlled. Pickett and colleagues[28] reported the incidence of surgical complications from cervical arthroplasty with the Bryan cervical disk arthroplasty that included hematoma evacuation (1%), radiculopathy/myelopathy (4%), and dysphagia/dysphonia (4%).[28] Current reported incidence of radiculopathy or peripheral nerve

injury with anterior cervical spine surgery ranges from 0.2% to 3.2%.[28–30] Airway compromise during the postoperative period from hematoma or edema has a reported incidence of 1.7% to 6.0%.[29–31]

Common postoperative hurdles with anterior cervical surgery are dysphagia and dysphonia. Factors associated with difficulty swallowing or hoarseness postoperatively are multifactorial and are described in the literature in association with anterior cervical fusion.[32] The incidence has been reported as high as 28% to 57%[32–35] with some degree of dysphagia postoperatively and concerns of symptoms underreported.[32] Lower dysphagia rates have been reported with arthroplasty.[36,37] Datta and colleagues[36] evaluated 45 patients who underwent ProDisc-C arthroplasty and 44 patients who underwent an ACDF with plate fixation. Follow-up demonstrated dysphagic complaints of 2.2% and 4.5% in the arthroplasty and fusion groups, respectively. Furthermore, prospective randomized clinical studies have also reported improved long-term dysphasia resolution with arthroplasty.[37] The use of self-retaining retractors causing sustained pressure on the esophagus may promote postoperative systems and use of handheld retractors is encouraged. Tortolani and colleagues[38] analyzed the intraesophageal pressures during anterior cervical plating and disk arthroplasty in a cadaveric study. They concluded that the insertion of a cervical TDR requires less esophageal retraction and therefore reduced intraesophageal pressure than anterior cervical plating.

INDICATIONS AND CONTRAINDICATIONS

Indications and contraindications to TDR have been identified and established as probable causes of failure and complications if not adhered to.[11,12] Cervical TDR indications include radiculopathy or myelopathy caused by 1 or 2 levels of cervical stenosis or compression with or without axial neck pain.[12,39–41] These criteria are similar to those for ACDF and include disk herniation pathology and spondylosis. After adequate decompression is obtained, the implant is used to restore intervertebral disk height, neuroforaminal height, and overall cervical sagittal and coronal alignment. Severe spondylosis, including bridging osteophytes and hypertrophic spondylarthrosis, are contraindications to TDR. These disease pathologies preclude the required motion and disk height of 2° and 50%, respectively.[41] **Table 2** provides a summary of the indications and contraindications for cervical TDR from the FDA IDE Trials.

Table 2
Cervical total disk replacement contraindications and indications

Indications	Contraindications
Pathology involving levels C3 to T1	Isolated axial neck pain
Cervical degenerative disk disease or signs of radiculopathy or myelopathy with or without axial neck pain	Ankylosing spondylitis Pregnancy
Disk herniation with radiculopathy/myelopathy	Rheumatoid arthritis, autoimmune disease
Spondylotic radiculopathy/myelopathy	Diffuse idiopathic skeletal hyperostosis
Above pathology and symptoms failing conservative treatment (weakness, paresthesias, radicular pain, hyperactive reflexes, abnormal sensation)	Severe spondylosis, bridging osteophytes, ossification of the posterior longitudinal ligament Metal allergy to implant materials Disk height loss >50%
	3 or More vertebral levels requiring treatment
	Spinal infection, active malignancy
	Systemic disease, insulin dependant diabetes mellitus, HIV, hepatitis B/C
	Metabolic bone disease, osteoporosis/osteopenia Trauma
	Morbid obesity, body mass index >40
	Absence of motion <2°
	Instability, translation >3 mm, >11° Rotational difference between adjacent levels

Data from McAfee PC. The indications for lumbar and cervical disc replacement. Spine J 2004;4:177S–81S; and Auerbach JD, Kristofer JJ, Christian IF, et al. The prevalence of indications and contraindications to cervical total disc replacement. Spine J 2008;8:711–6.

IMPLANT FAILURE—SURGICAL CASE COMPLICATIONS

Success of cervical disk arthroplasty is related to proper patient selection, surgical indications, and technique. **Table 3** lists the types of failures of TDRs. As discussed previously, the completion of long-term studies is paramount in revealing common methods of implant failure. Implant failure in the absence of surgical technical error is an uncommon occurrence.

Polyethylene core fractures, dislocations (**Fig. 2**), bearing surface wear, and implant breakage are all possibilities of failure. Currently the most obvious type of failure found on follow-up imaging is subtle implant migration and loosening, the majority of which is asymptomatic. Migration and loosening commonly result from poor implant sizing intraoperatively. Biologic causes can also result in loosening with poor ingrowth, end plate resorption, and subsidence. Vertebral body fracture has also been reported and may cause implant loosening. Its occurrence in the literature has been correlated with implant design and surgical technique[42–44] but it is also associated with trauma (**Fig. 3**). It is commonly

reported in multiple-level TDR with implants utilizing keel fixation. The mechanisms of fracture can result from shallow keel cuts, implant design, dull instrumentation, crack propagation, and lack

Table 3
Summary of total disk replacement failure types

Type	Example
Implant failure	Bearing surface failure
Iatrogenic deformity	Scoliosis "kyphosis"
Bone-implant interface failure	Migration Subsidence Dislodgement Vertebral body fracture
Host response	Heterotopic ossification Osteolysis
Infection	
Supraphysiologic motion	

Data from McAfee PC, Gloystein D, Cunningham BW. Failed disc replacement. In: Herkowitz HN, Garfin SR, Eismon FJ, et al, editors. Rothman-Simeone the spine, vol. II. Philadelphia: Elsevier; 2011. p. 1825–39.

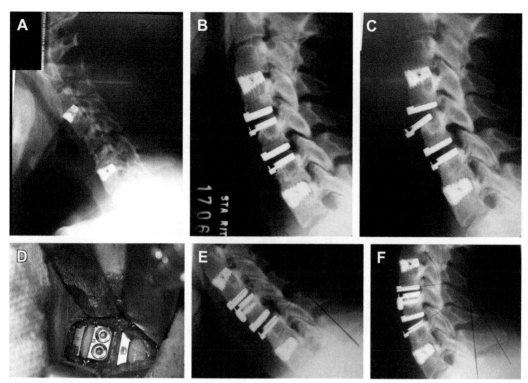

Fig. 2. (*A*) A 39-year-old woman who had previously undergone a cervical arthrodesis procedure at C3-C4 and C6-C7. Unfortunately she was locked in a kyphotic alignment with herniated disks at both intermediate levels (C4-C5 and C5-C6). She presented with bilateral radicular pain and neck pain. (*B*) PCM cervical disk (NuVasive Inc, San Diego, CA, USA) arthroplasty at C4-C5 and C5-C6 with anterior soft tissue releases. Kyphosis was corrected with resolved radicular and neck pain. (*C*) At 5 months postoperatively, patient had a severe fall that dislodged the caudal component in the C4-C5 interspace. In retrospect, there had not been sufficient bony support under the prosthesis at the anterior-superior corner of C5 vertebra body. (*D*) Intraoperative image demonstrating supplementation of the inferior component of the C4-C5 level with 2 screws and an anterior prosthetic flange. (*E*) Postoperative flexion radiograph documents stability at both C4-C5 and C5-C6 implant levels. (*F*) Postoperative extension radiographs demonstrates 26° of flexion-extension mobility at both prosthetic levels, which was the identical range of motion after the primary disk replacement procedures.

of finesse during final implant placement. Subsidence may also result from fracture to the vertebral end plate during insertion. If the keel cuts are too shallow, attempts at impacting the implant into the optimal position can bottom out the keel and fracture the vertebral body.

Local response to implant placement can result in heterotopic ossification or inflammation. Heller and colleagues[45] reported that ossification occurs in the first 100 days following surgery and nonsteroidal anti-inflammatory drugs should be implemented in high-risk patients. Its formation defeats the purpose of placing a motion-preserving device and precautions should be taken accordingly. Few studies have been completed on disk arthroplasty wear debris production and its corresponding effects. Results have shown minimal debris and minimal inflammatory response.[46] Also, the limited range of motion

within the spine compared with other joint replacement implants reduces the volumetric wear of the implant. Although wear particles generated are considered minimal, there are still concerns with its overall affect. Metal hypersensitivity has caused pseudotumor formation from metal-on-metal combalt-chrome prosthesis implants.[47]

With multilevel TDR, there is a risk of segmental kyphosis deformity postoperatively and its occurrence has been reported in the literature.[48–50] Loss of preoperative cervical lordosis has been reported in up to 49% of patients treated with cervical arthroplasty.[28] Concerns that this complication may affect not only the biomechanical function of the cervical TDR implant but also the adjacent levels. Abnormal stresses on the paraspinal musculature and axial cervical spine may result in discomfort and pain. The sagittal plane deformity has been attributed to different sources.

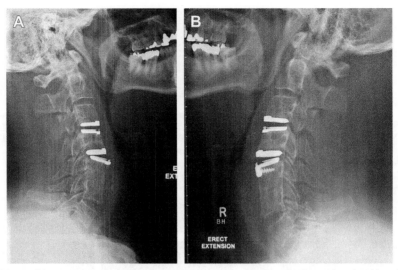

Fig. 3. (*A*) A 50-year-old man 6 months after a 2-level PCM cervical arthroplasty was involved in a head-on motor vehicle collision. The lateral radiograph demonstrates a fracture of the superior end plate of C5 causing an acute loosening of the lower component of the C4-C5 prosthesis. (*B*) Revision surgery of the loose low-profile component with a revision PCM component incorporating a flange and 2 anchoring screws. The patient had an uneventful recovery and had restoration of cervical range of motion to the same preinjury levels. (Surgery performed by Matthew Scott Young.)

Careful attention to surgical technique and optimal implant placement reduces postoperatively deformity (**Fig. 4**). Implant positioning must not be off-axis and should be aligned accordingly to the global alignment of the cervical spine. Intraoperative factors also include angle of prosthesis insertion, prosthesis length, loss of preoperative disk space height, and appropriate end plate preparation. Performing a complete diskectomy and visualization of the disk space are important for end plate preparation. This not only allows for appropriate visualization but adequate decompression. Decompression should be performed far enough laterally to decompress the spinal cord and nerve roots but not so far laterally to endanger the vertebral arteries. The use of a high-speed burr is not recommended until the diskectomy is completed. Early usage of the burr without adequate visualization of the disk space may result in removing excessive bone stock and disruption of the end plates. Most of the decompression and bone removal can be accomplished safely with a Kerrison rongeur and curettes. Incomplete decompression at this stage leads to recurrent or new radiculopathy. Once the end plates are adequately visualized, implant base-plate and vertical dimension fit can be addressed. Coverage of the end plates should be obtained with the largest size implant that allows proper seating along the periphery of the vertebral body. Undersized implants increase stress concentrations per unit area and increase the propensity to subside.[51] The bone at the periphery of the end plate is the strongest and prevents subsidence. In regards to the vertical dimension, overdistracting the disk space should be avoided. The overall implant height should create a disk height similar to that of an adjacent normal segment.

Patients should be evaluated for facet disease from both clinical and radiographic perspectives before undergoing a cervical TDR. This evaluation should be completed at both the operative level and at adjacent levels. Unlike an ACDF where a fusion prevents motion at painful facet joints, a TDR allows motion at these joints and possibly worsens the facet disease and discomfort. Facet pathology may also arise from oversized or undersized implants that lead to alterations in the biomechanical kinematics of the posterior elements. Persistent neck pain has been reported after cervical arthroplasty[28] and could be the result of underlying facet pathology.

Implant positioning is dictated by spinal balance and overall alignment of the cervical spine. Lordosis is important for maintenance of normal kinematics and should match the patient's global cervical alignment. The implant's posterior edge should correspond with the posterior edge of the vertebral body. It is here that the center of rotation of most implant designs correlate with the natural center of rotation of the spine.[52] Malpositioning of the implant and undersizing can lead to

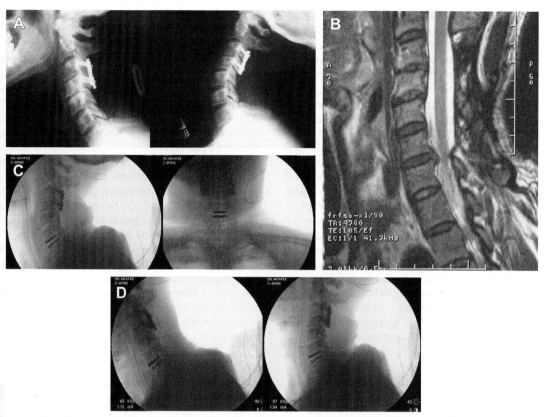

Fig. 4. (*A*) A 43-year-old man presented with a large herniated disk at C6-C7 but had previously undergone wide laminectomies from C3 to the middle of C7. (*B*) MRI illustrates a large right-sided herniated nucleus pulposus that corresponded to right triceps weakness and numbness in the right C7 dermatome. (*C*) The patient was treated with an anterior diskectomy and PCM cervical arthroplasty at C6-C7. (*D*) Intraoperative flexion extension stability was documented by direct manipulation under fluoroscopic visualization without rocking or subluxation of the prosthetic components. Radiographs documented 9° of flexion-extension motion. The patient's symptoms resolved and he was able to return to unrestricted work in 6 weeks. At 5 years postoperatively, he continues to be neurologically intact without any symptoms or further pathology.

asymmetric loading of the cervical spine in the coronal plane. This asymmetry results in a decreased foramen dimension on one side and a recurrence of radiculopathy from the bony foraminal stenosis.[53] On physical examination, a reduction of symptoms may be seen with lateral bending toward the offset side of the device. Fluoroscopy can be used intraoperatively to identify the midline of the vertebral bodies. This landmark should be used in preparation of the end plates and vertebral body to avoid straying lateral. Midline orientation can also be verified with visualization of the uncovertebral joints.

Infection surrounding the cervical disk implant is not a common complication. Knowledge of treatment of infected arthroplasty systems comes from the total joint replacement literature. In the acute setting, attempts at treating an infected TDR with antibiotics alone can lead to progressive bone destruction and morbidity. Revision to fusion

should follow clinical signs of infection as a salvage procedure.

As with any revision, the risks and complications associated with the approach are increased. Unlike anterior lumbar revision procedures, cervical arthroplasty revisions have a much lower risk through the same surgical approach.[54] Revision through the anterior exposure at less than 2 weeks postoperatively can be completed with little additional morbidity because adhesion formation is minimal. At this time there should be a low threshold to revise implants that show evidence of early failure or complications. Approach through the contralateral side in a scar-free plane is an option as well, but occult vocal cord paralysis must be ruled out before the planned approach. Preoperative planning must be completed and is critical for successful outcomes. The cause of failure of the TDR procedure must be identified and surgical treatment tailored specifically to that established mode of failure. Intraoperative findings consisting of vertebral body fracture, bone loss, deformity, or instability should be revised to an interbody arthrodesis. A common mistake with revision disk replacements is overstuffing of the disk space in an attempt to reduce risks of migration. The implant in this situation acts like an arthrodesis cage and is not optimal for motion preservation. Furthermore, during revision surgery too much bone may be removed with removal of the end plates. This results in subsidence of the prosthesis if revised to a TDR; therefore, an anterior fusion is preferred. Patients must be counseled on possible changes to the original surgical plan if complications arise intraoperatively. A posterior approach should be used for patients with a strong contraindication for repeat anterior cervical surgery and without the necessity of implant removal. The need to revise from a posterior approach is rare and carries its own risks and in the authors' experience should be avoided. Additional posterior stability is required in the setting of signification subsidence and kyphosis with implant removal.

The complexity of cervical TDR replacement with distracting pin positioning, rasping, spacers, and prosthetic trails requires the use of intraoperative fluoroscopy. This is especially important with revision surgery, and orientation must be confirmed with radiographs. This requires more than conventional radiographs; thus, the patient and room equipment must be positioned so that fluoroscopic images can be obtained. Patients should be placed in the supine position on a radiolucent operating table. The cervical spine must be aligned in a neutral posture. The surgical incision can be made in a transverse or oblique fashion over the corresponding cervical spine levels. These levels can be identified via palpation or with radiographic evaluation. The dissection is continued to the superficial fascia containing the platysma, it is important to preserve this muscle for a layered closure in revision cases. Additionally, during arthroplasty procedures, the patient's head should not be taped down or restricted. After insertion of the TDR trial or prosthesis, the anesthesiologist can take the neck through a range of

---

Box 1
Cervical total disk replacement key points

1. Cervical TDR can preserve motion at adjacent segments and avoid limitations associated with ACDF, including
   a. Bone graft site morbidity
   b. Adjacent segment disease associated with cervical fusion
   c. Pseudarthrosis
   d. Anterior cervical plating
2. Failure to identify the surgical indications/contraindications for TDR may lead to higher clinical failure rates.
3. Implant size and position intraoperatively should be adjusted according to
   a. Coverage of the vertebral body peripheral end plate
   b. Cervical spine alignment and lordosis
   c. Disc space height and avoiding overdistraction
4. Avoid asymmetric orientation of the implant:
   a. Identify the midline and avoid straying from this when preparing the vertebral body.
   b. The implant should be positioned in the corresponding center of the disk space on the anterior-posterior radiographs.
5. Revision surgery for failed TDR may preclude subsequent revision to TDR. Indications and contraindications should be reviewed during the preoperative planning. Anterior spinal fusion is the revision strategy of choice for pathology, involving
   a. Poor bone quality and quantity
   b. Infection
   c. Cervical instability
   d. Cervical deformity

motion with fluoroscopic visualization. This allows the surgeon to insure that components do not rock or impinge at any point along the full flexion-extension arc.

SUMMARY

Clinical results are encouraging and have shown comparable results between TDR and fusion. As biomechanical studies have shown, maintaining motion and preventing adjacent segment degeneration are the main driving factors of cervical arthroplasty. Procedural complications associated with an anterior cervical fusion can also be avoided with cervical disk arthroplasty. Long-term clinical results will help identify the role of TDR in the treatment of cervical spine pathology. Although intermediate-term clinical results are promising, failures and complications will emerge as implant usage becomes more prevalent. This is illustrated by the reports of pseudotumor formation inside the cervical canal due to metal hypersensitivity and exuberant inflammatory response to metal-on-metal prostheses; the true incidence of this complication is not currently known. Complications of cervical disk replacement can be associated with improper implant sizing, insertion, and surgical indications. Revision surgery should be directed at addressing the specific cause of implant failure and may not be amendable to a subsequent disk replacement but anterior fusion. The presence of poor bone quality, deformity, and instability precludes revision to a TDR. **Box 1** provides a review and summary of key points.

REFERENCES

1. Bohlman HH, Emery SE, Goodfellow DB, et al. Robinson anterior cervical diskectomy and arthrodesis for cervical radiculopathy, Long term follow-up of 122 patients. J Bone Joint Surg Am 1993;75: 1298–307.
2. Robinson RA, Smith G. Anterolateral cervical disk removal and interbody fusion for cervical disk syndrome. Bull Johns Hopkins Hosp 1955;96:223–4.
3. Eck JC, Humphreys SC, Lim TH, et al. Biomechanical study on the effect of cervical spine fusion on adjacent-level intradiscal pressure and segmental motion. Spine 2002;27:2431–4.
4. DiAngelo DJ, Robertson JT, Metcalf NH, et al. Biomechanical testing of an artificial cervical joint and an anterior cervical plate. J Spinal Disord Tech 2003;16:314–23.
5. Maiman DJ, Kumaresan S, Yoganandan N, et al. Biomechanical effect of anterior cervical spine fusion on adjacent segments. Biomed Mater Eng 1999;9(1):27–38.
6. Wigfield CC, Skrzypiec D, Jackowski A, et al. Internal stress distribution in cervical intervertebral discs: the influence of an artificial cervical joint and simulated anterior interbody fusion. J Spinal Disord Tech 2003;16:44–9.
7. Hilibrand AS, Carlson GD, Palumbo MA, et al. Radiculopathy and myelopathy at segments adjacent to the site of a previous anterior cervical arthrodesis. J Bone Joint Surg Am 1999;81:519–28.
8. Deyo RA, Nachemson A, Mirza SK. Spinal-fusion surgery the case for restraint. N Engl J Med 2004; 350:722–6.
9. Lipson SJ. Spinal fusion surgery: advances and concerns. N Engl J Med 2004;350(7):643–4.
10. Phillips FM, Carlson G, Emery SE, et al. Anterior cervical pseudarthrosis. Natural history and treatment. Spine 1997;22:1585–9.
11. McAfee PC, Gloystein D, Cunningham BW. Failed disc replacement. In: Herkowitz HN, Garfin SR, Eismon FJ, et al, editors. Rothman-Simeone the spine, vol. II. Philadelphia: Elsevier; 2011. p. 1825–39.
12. McAfee PC. The indications for lumbar and cervical disc replacement. Spine J 2004;4:177S–81S.
13. Goffin J, Van Calenbergh F, Van Loon J, et al. Intermediate follow-up after treatment of degenerative disc disease with the Bryan Cervical Disc Prosthesis: single-level and bi-level. Spine 2003;28(24):2673–8.
14. Bertagnoli R, Yue JJ, Pfeiffer F, et al. Early results after Pro Disc-C cervical disc replacement. J Neurosurg Spine 2005;2(4):403–10.
15. Pimenta L, McAfee P, Cappuccino A, et al. Clinical experience with the new artificial cervical PCM (Cervitech) disc. Spine J 2004;4(6):315–21.
16. Fuller DA, Kirkpatrick JS, Emery SE, et al. A kinematic Study of the cervical spine before and after segmental arthrodesis. Spine 1998;23:1649–56.
17. Goffin J, Geusens E, Vantomme N, et al. Long-term follow-up after interbody fusion of the cervical spine. J Spinal Disord Tech 2004;17:79–85.
18. Garrido BJ, Wilhite J, Nakano M, et al. Adjacent level cervical ossification after Bryan cervical disc arthroplasty compared with anterior cervical discectomy and fusion. J Bone Joint Surg Am 2011;93(13):1185–9.
19. Brown CA, Eismont FJ. Complications in spinal fusion. Orthop Clin North Am 1998;29:679–99.
20. Sandhu HS, Grewal HS, Parvataneni H. Bone grafting for spinal fusion. Orthop Clin North Am 1999; 30:685–98.
21. Summers BN, Eisenstein SM. Donor Site pain from ilium: a complication of lumbar spine fusion. J Bone Joint Surg Br 1989;71:677–80.
22. Buttermann GR. Prospective nonrandomized comparison of an allograft with bone morphogenic protein versus an iliac-crest autograft in anterior cervical diskectomy and fusion. Spine J 2008;8:426–35.
23. Brown MD, Malinin TI, Davis PB. A roentgenographic evaluation of frozen allografts versus

autografts in anterior cervical spine fusions. Clin Orthop Relat Res 1976;119:231–6.

24. Bishop RC, Moore KA, Hadley MN. Anterior cervical interbody fusion using autogeneic and allogeneic bone graft substrate: a prospective comparative analysis. J Neurosurg 1996;85:206–10.

25. Floyd T, Ohnmeiss D. A meta-analysis of autograft versus allograft in anterior cervical fusion. Eur Spine J 2000;9:398–403.

26. Suchomel P, Barsa P, Buchvald P, et al. Autologous versus allogenic bone grafts in instrumented anterior-cervical discectomy and fusion: a prospective study with respect to bone union pattern. Eur Spine J 2004;13:510–5.

27. Malloy KM, Hilibrand AS. Autograft versus allograft in degenerative cervical disease. Clin Orthop Relat Res 2002;394:27–38.

28. Pickett GE, Sekhon LH, Sears WR, et al. Complications with cervical arthroplasty. J Neurosurg Spine 2006;4:98–105.

29. Emery SE, Bohlman HH, Bolesta MJ, et al. Anterior Cervical Decompression and arthrodesis for the treatment of cervical spondylotic myelopathy. Two to seventeen-year follow-up. J Bone Joint Surg Am 1998;80:941–51.

30. Epstein NE, Hollingsworth R, Nardi D, et al. Can airway complications following multilevel anterior cervical surgery be avoided? J Neurosurg 2001; 94:185–8.

31. Sagi HC, Beutler W, Carroll E, et al. Airway compications associated with surgery on the anterior cervical spine. Spine 2002;27:949–53.

32. Smith-Hammond CA, New KC, Pietrobon R, et al. Prospective analysis of incidence and risk factors of dysphagia in spine surgery patients: Comparison of anterior cervical, posterior cervical, and lumbar procedures. Spine 2004;29:1441–6.

33. Edwards CC II, Karpitskaya Y, Cha C, et al. Accurate identification of adverse outcomes after cervical spine surgery. J Bone Joint Surg Am 2004;86:251–6.

34. Lee MJ, Bazaz R, Furey CG, et al. Risk factors for dysphagia after anterior cervical spine surgery: a two-year prospective cohort study. Spine J 2007; 7:141–7.

35. Lee MJ, Bazaz R, Furey CG, et al. Influence of anterior cervical plate design on dysphagia: a 2-year prospective longitudinal follow-up study. J Spinal Disord Tech 2005;18:406–9.

36. Datta J, Janssen M, Murry D, et al. Incidence of dysphagia comparing cervical arthroplasty and ACDF with internal fixation. Spine J 2006;6:97.

37. McAfee PC, Cappuccion A, DeVine J, et al. Lower incidence of dysphagia with cervical arthroplasty compared to ACDF in a prospective randomized clinical trials. Spine J 2008;8:43S–4S.

38. Tortolani JP, Cunningham BW, Vigna F, et al. A comparison of retraction pressures during anterior cervical plate surgery and cervical disc replacement: a cadaveric study. J Spinal Disord Tech 2006;19(5):312–7.

39. Anderson PA, Rosler DM, Rouleau JP, et al. Evaluation of the inflammatory response to the Bryan Cervical Disc Prosthesis in a caprine model. Eur Spine J 2002;11:S36.

40. Bryan VE. Cervical motion segment replacement. Eur Spine J 2002;11:S92–7.

41. Auerbach JD, Kristofer JJ, Christian IF, et al. The prevalence of indications and contraindications to cervical total disc replacement. Spine J 2008;8: 711–6.

42. Datta JC, Janssen ME, Beckham R, et al. Sagittal split fractures in multilevel cervical arthroplasty using keeled prosthesis. J Spinal Disord Tech 2007;20(1):89–92.

43. Shim CS, Lee S, Maeng DH, et al. Vertical split fracture of the vertebral body following total disc replacement using ProDisc: report of two cases. J Spinal Disord Tech 2005;18:465–9.

44. Shim CS, Shin HD, Lee SH. Posterior avulsion fracture at an adjacent vertebral body during cervical disc replacement with ProDisc-C: a case report. J Spinal Disord Tech 2007;20(6):568–72.

45. Heller JG, Park AE, Tortolani PJ, et al. Computed tomography (CT) scan assessment of paravertebral bone after total cervical disc replacement: temporal relationships and the effect of NSAIDs. Read at the Annual Meeting of the Cervical Spine Research Society, European Section; 2003. Barcelona, Spain, June 19–20, 2003.

46. Hu N, Cunningham BW, McAfee PC, et al. Porous coated motion cervical disc replacement: a biomechanical, histomorphometric, and biologic wear analysis in a caprine model. Spine 2006;31(15): 1666–73.

47. Buchowski JM, Sekhon LH, Yoon DH, et al. Adverse events of cervical arthroplasty. Tech Orthop 2010; 25(2):138–44.

48. Fong SY, Du Plessis SJ, Casha S, et al. Design limitations of Bryan disc arthroplasty. Spine 2006;6: 233–41.

49. Pickett GE, Rouleau JP, Duggal N. Kinematic analysis of the cervical spine following implantation of an artificial cervical disc. Spine 2005;30: 1949–54.

50. Shim CS, Lee SH, Park HJ, et al. Early clinical and radiologic outcomes of cervical arthroplasty with Bryan Cervical Disc prosthesis. J Spinal Disord Tech 2006;19:465–70.

51. Lin C, Kank H, Rouleau JP, et al. Stress analysis of the interface between cervical vertebrae end plates and the Bryan, Prestige LP, Prodisc-C disc

prostheses: an in vivo image-based finite element study. Spine 2009;34:1554–60.

52. Ishii T, Mukai Y, Hosono N, et al. Kinematics of the subaxial cervical spine in rotation: in vivo three-dimensional analysis. Spine 2006;31:155–60.

53. Goffin J. Complications of cervical disc arthroplasty. Semin Spine Surg 2006;18:87–98.

54. Sekhon LH. Reversal of anterior cervical fusion with a cervical arthroplasty prosthesis. J Spinal Disord Tech 2005;18:S125–8.

Surgical Management of Complex Spinal Deformity

Melissa M. Erickson, MD[a], Bradford L. Currier, MD[b],*

KEYWORDS

- Surgical management • Complex spinal deformity
- Cervical deformity

Surgical treatment of complex cervical spinal deformities can be challenging operations. Patients often present with debilitating conditions ranging from generalized decreased quality of life to quadriplegia. Surgical treatment can be divided into anterior, posterior, or combined procedures. A thorough understanding of anatomy, pathology, and treatment options is necessary. This article focuses on the surgical treatment of complex spinal deformity.

PRESENTATION

Most commonly, patients present with cervical deformity as a chronic finding. Deformity may be incidentally found during the work-up of other congenital cardiac, renal, or intraspinal malformations.[1] Patients can present with a spectrum of physical complaints, including neck pain, radiculopathy, myelopathy, and cosmetic dissatisfaction. Neurologic deficits can be caused by central stenosis leading to myelopathy or foraminal stenosis leading to radiculopathy. The spinal cord can also be draped over the apex of a bony defect and become tethered by the dentate ligaments in what has been described as the bowstring effect. This condition can lead to chronic changes in the microvascular circulation of the cord, resulting in spinal cord atrophy or myelomalacia.[2] Patients may have complex radiculopathic complaints that can be unilateral or bilateral. Pain can radiate into the anterior chest, neck, or periscapular area. Patients typically have distal paresthesias and proximal arm pain (**Fig. 1**).[3]

Patients may present with acute deformity secondary to trauma. If patients have a chronic deformity from ankylosis of the cervical spine and experience sudden neck pain, a fracture is presumed until proven otherwise. These fractures are often 3-column injuries that are grossly unstable and can result in complete quadriplegia.

Kyphosis can adversely affect forward gaze, swallowing, and breathing. It can also result in compensatory lumbar hyperlordosis and associated low back pain. Cervical kyphosis causes the posterior musculature to be under constant contraction to maintain upright posture, contributing to neck pain.[2]

CAUSES

Complex cervical spine deformities can develop secondary to multiple causes. Degenerative disease usually causes symptoms that develop insidiously. Advanced degeneration can alter the normal biomechanics of the spine. The weight-bearing axis is translated anteriorly as the disk spaces decrease in height, leading to tensile load in the posterior elements. Ligaments become attenuated, and the progression of kyphotic deformity ensues.[4]

Iatrogenic deformity is most commonly caused by surgeries that were performed to treat uncomplicated neurologic symptoms.[2] Postoperative kyphosis has been reported after anterior-based surgeries, such as anterior cervical discectomy without fusion, anterior cervical discectomy and fusion (ACDF) without plating, ACDF with stand-alone cages, and corpectomies without posterior

[a] Mayo Clinic College of Medicine, Mayo Clinic, 200 First Street Southwest, Rochester, MN 55905, USA
[b] Department of Orthopedic Surgery, Mayo Clinic College of Medicine, Mayo Clinic, 200 First Street Southwest, Rochester, MN 55905, USA
* Corresponding author.
E-mail address: currier.bradford@mayo.edu

Orthop Clin N Am 43 (2012) 109–122
doi:10.1016/j.ocl.2011.10.001

instrumentation.[5-8] Posteriorly, an excessive facetectomy can result in segmental instability that results in kyphosis. The incidence of postlaminectomy kyphosis has been reported to be as high as 21%.[9] Younger age at the time of surgery, 4 or more laminectomy levels, laminectomy performed in conjunction with facetectomy, increased preoperative range of motion, and surgery involving the C2 lamina and its attachments have been shown to be risk factors. Suk and colleagues[10] described

postlaminoplasty kyphosis occurring in 10.6% of patients with an average of 12° kyphosis.

Inflammatory disorders that commonly involve the cervical spine include rheumatoid arthritis (RA) and ankylosing spondylitis (AS). RA affects 0.3% to 1.5% of the population. Despite the improved medical management of RA, cervical spine manifestations occur in up to 86% of patients.[11] Atlantoaxial instability, basilar invagination, subaxial subluxation, and combinations of

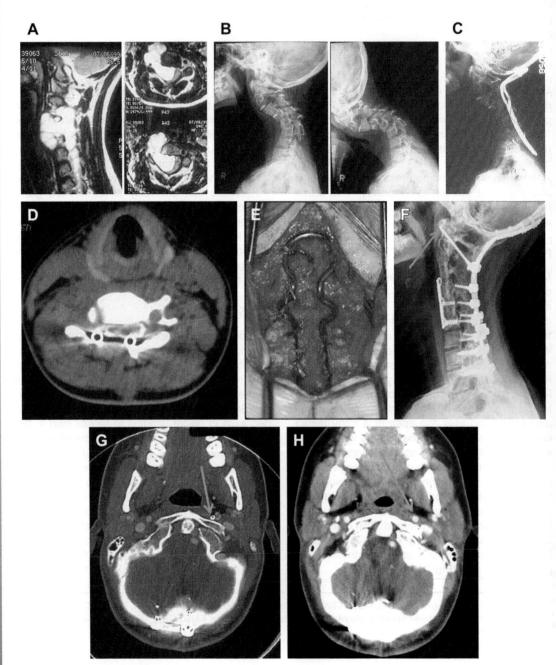

the 3 can occur (**Fig. 2**A–D). AS is a debilitating inflammatory disorder. Bony syndesmophytes form across disk spaces. Early in the disease, facet joints are affected and patients tend to flex their spine to unload the facets. This state can ultimately lead to the classic chin-on-chest deformity.

Dropped head deformity (DHD) is a severe, flexible, cervicothoracic kyphosis caused by weakness of the neck extensor muscles. Primary DHD may be caused by a systemic neuromuscular disease, including myasthenia gravis, amyotrophic lateral sclerosis (ALS), congenital myopathy, chronic inflammatory polyneuropathy, and polymyositis, or an extrapyramidal disease (Parkinson disease). Primary DHD may also be caused by an isolated local condition, such as inflammatory myositis and dystonia. Secondary causes of DHD include prior treatment with radiotherapy and local botulinum toxin injection (**Fig. 3**A–D).[12]

EVALUATION

All patients should have a thorough clinical and radiographic evaluation. When obtaining the history, special attention is given to details that may elucidate underlying causes and factors that may alter the treatment plan or prognosis. Dystonia can affect biomechanical muscle balance and may put patients at an increased risk of recurrence. History of radiation therapy may put patients at a higher risk of wound healing.

Swallowing dysfunction may worsen postoperatively and impact nutritional status.

Physical examination should be thorough. Soft tissues surrounding the spine should be assessed, especially in patients who have had prior radiation or surgery. If soft tissue is tenuous, a plastic surgery consult can be obtained preoperatively. The chin-brow to vertical angle should be assessed by measuring the angle between a line from the brow to the chin and a vertical line when patients stand with the hips and knees extended with the neck in neutral. Suk and colleagues[13] found that patients that underwent correction to a chin-brow vertical angle ranging from -10° to 10° had better horizontal gaze. Overall sagittal alignment should be assessed with knees extended because patients will often crouch at the knees to maintain horizontal gaze or overall balance. Posterior musculature should be inspected for tone. Patients should also be examined lying supine. The chin-brow tohorizontal angle should be measured as well as the distance the occiput to the bed to assess the flexibility of the condition.

A complete spine examination can help localize the lesion. Central stenosis tends to have findings consistent with myelopathy. Foraminal stenosis can present with radiculopathy. Many patients will have mixed findings.

Plain films are used to assess the deformity and identify any congenital anomalies, prior fusions, and previously placed instrumentation. Flexion and extension films are used to determine

---

Fig. 1. A 12-year-old girl with a chordoma at C2 and 3 was referred following intralesional anteroposterior resection and motion-sparing reconstruction elsewhere. She had a laminoplasty posteriorly and placement of nonstructural graft and mesh at C2-4 anteriorly following her tumor resection. She developed a progressive swan-neck deformity, and her surgeon attempted a posterior occipital-cervical fusion with a Ransford loop (ISrugicraft, UK). She developed a pseudoarthrosis, and the rods migrated into her spinal canal. She was eventually referred for complaints of cervical deformity, pain, and myelopathy. She underwent a multistage reconstruction as follows: stage I: posterior removal of rods with decompression and osteotomies through the partially fused facet joints; stage II: cervical traction for 5 days; stage III: anterior decompression and fusion with 2 grafts and kick plate; stage IV (same day as stage III): posterior O-C fusion with rod/screw construct with iliac crest autograft. She subsequently underwent proton beam radiation therapy for tumor control. The tip of the single transarticular screw used during the reconstruction was found to be compressing the internal carotid artery. It was removed without sequelae, and she is disease free and functioning well with minimal pain and no neurologic deficit 12 years following her tumor resection. (A) Sagittal and axial MRI images showing the chordoma before resection elsewhere. (B) Sequential lateral radiographs showing progressive swan-neck deformity following her tumor resection and motion-sparing reconstruction. (C) Lateral radiograph at presentation with progressive deformity, pain, myelopathy, and pseudoarthrosis. (D) CT myelogram image of C5-6 at presentation showing Ransford loop has migrated into the spinal canal causing cord compression. (E) Clinical photograph taken during stage I showing Ransford loop has migrated into the spinal canal. Fibrous tissue within the subaxial facet joints was removed to loosen up the spine in preparation for traction. (F) Final lateral radiograph showing sagittal alignment has been restored and fusion is solid. Only one transarticular screw could be used because the tumor resection caused the posterior elements to be deficient. Subsequent evaluation before proton beam therapy (see Fig. 1[G]) showed that the tip of the transarticular screw (arrow) was found to be abutting and compressing the ipsilateral internal carotid artery. (G) CT with contrast showing the tip of the transarticular screw (arrow) is abutting and compressing the left internal carotid artery at the anterior arch of the atlas. (H) CT with contrast following removal of the transarticular shows that the internal carotid artery (arrow) was not damaged. The authors now recommend a CT with contrast before placing screws into the lateral mass of the atlas.

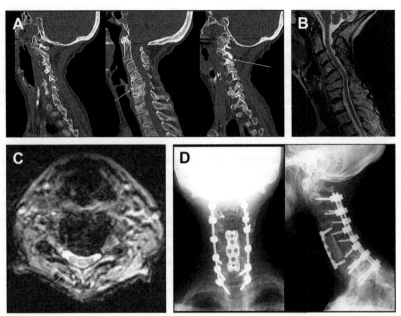

Fig. 2. A 63-year-old woman presented with complaints of progressive neck fatigue and deformity for 3 years. She had to hold her head up with her hand, otherwise her chin rested on her chest. She denied trauma but had fallen several times because of mild myelopathy. After a comprehensive evaluation, the cause of her DHD was thought to be posterior neck muscular weakness secondary to remote history of high-dose radiation therapy for Hodgkin disease. She underwent a 2-stage reconstruction. The first stage was done anteriorly because she had ankylosis of the C5-6 vertebral bodies, which was responsible for her fixed kyphosis, and she had no ankylosis of the facet joints. C5 and 6 corpectomies and allograft fibular strut graft fusion decompressed the stenosis and corrected the fixed deformity. The open facet joints permitted the reduction of the deformity from the front. C2-3, C3-4, and C7-T1 anterior cervical diskectomies and allograft fusions enhanced the overall fusion rate and helped prevent late loss of correction. Stage II was done several days later and involved an instrumented C2-T2 fusion to maintain correction and enhance the fusion rate. One and one-half years postoperatively, she had no loss of correction, no neurologic deficit, no neck or arm pain, and her range of motion was approximately 50% of normal. (*A*) Sagittal reformatted CT images show spontaneous fusion C5-6 with kyphotic deformity (*small arrow*). None of the cervical facet joints were ankylosed. The right C2-3 facet joint was eroded (*large arrow*). The C2-3 level was found to be hypermobile on flexion/extension films. Note that only the fixed component of her deformity is appreciated on her CT images. Clinically, she had a chin-on-chest deformity. (*B*) Lateral MRI demonstrating fixed kyphotic deformity with stenosis at C4-7. (*C*) Axial MRI at C5-6 demonstrating stenosis and cord deformity with high T2 signal in the cord (*arrow*). (*D*) Postoperative anteroposterior and lateral radiographs demonstrate the multilevel anterior and posterior decompression and fusion with restored alignment.

flexibility of the deformity and status of prior fusions. Full-length standing films with knees extended are used to assess global balance. Magnetic resonance imaging (MRI) assesses soft tissue and should be used to evaluate for spinal stenosis and evidence of cord atrophy or myelomalacia. A computed tomography (CT) scan with coronal and sagittal reconstructions should be obtained to further characterize bony anatomy. Prior surgical or congenital fusion can be more accurately evaluated with CT than plain radiographs. Pedicle morphology and the course of the vertebral arteries are noted. Adjacent joints are assessed for degeneration and spontaneous fusion. If patients have torticollis, a dynamic CT can be obtained to compare images taken with the patients' head turned maximally to each side to determine the mobility of the atlantoaxial joints. Contrast is used to assess the internal carotid arteries and vertebral arteries when upper cervical fusion is planned. Electromyography (EMG) can be used to localize radiculopathy and differentiate it from any peripheral neuropathy, shoulder complaints or referred pain.

Laboratory work-up includes standard preoperative laboratory tests. Any abnormalities in coagulation should be corrected preoperatively because blood loss can be significant, especially in revision cases. Nutritional and nicotine laboratory tests may be helpful to avoid problems with soft tissue healing and fusion. Blood tests that can screen for underlying myopathy include creatine kinase,

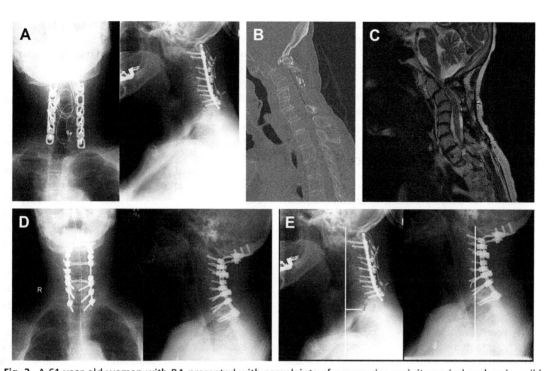

Fig. 3. A 61-year-old woman with RA presented with complaints of progressive occipitocervical neck pain, mild myelopathic symptoms, and kyphotic deformity. Ten years previously, she had undergone a C2-7 posterior decompression and fusion elsewhere. The authors were prepared to do a multistage procedure, with traction between stages as needed, but were able to achieve their goals with a single-stage posterior procedure. She had the instrumentation removed C2-7, laminectomies C1-4, osteotomies C2-3, C3-4, C4-5, and an occiput-T2 posterior fusion with a rod/screw construct and iliac crest bone graft. Following the decompression, the dura was kinked at the craniocervical junction, but an intraoperative ultrasound demonstrated good dural pulsation and CSF surrounding the spinal cord, so a duraplasty was not necessary. (*A*) Anteroposterior and lateral radiographs show prior laminectomies C5 and C6 and nonrigid posterior instrumentation C2-7. She has kyphosis C2-5, tilt to the right in the coronal plane, and cranial settling with impingement of the right-sided plate on the occiput. (*B*) Sagittal CT reformatted image shows cranial settling; the eroded tip of the odontoid has migrated into the foramen magnum. There is C1-2 subluxation with severe stenosis at the craniocervical junction. Other cuts showed occipitalization of C1. The spine is subluxed anteriorly at C2-3 and C3-4 and the spine is kyphotic from C2 to C5. The prior laminectomies of C5 and C6 are also seen. (*C*) Sagittal T2-weighted MRI demonstrates stenosis from the foramen magnum to C4. The stenosis is severe at the craniocervical junction. (*D*) Postoperative AP and lateral radiographs demonstrate improved alignment and stability following occipit-T2 fusion. (*E*) Preoperative (*left*) and postoperative (*right*) lateral radiographs demonstrate improved alignment. The spine is still kyphotic C2-4, but the global alignment is good and her head position allows comfortable forward gaze. A plumb line from the center of the foramen magnum now falls inside the C7 vertebral body.

aldolase, aspartate aminotransferase, alanine aminotransferase, and lactate dehydrogenase.

Patients often have multiple medical problems that can affect outcomes. Consideration should be given to obtaining preoperative consultations to optimize patient conditions before surgery. Neurology can rule out reversible causes of dystonia or other causes of neurologic deficits, such as peripheral neuropathy, multiple sclerosis, or ALS. Patients with previous anterior surgery should be evaluated by an ear, nose, and throat (ENT) specialist. Vocal cords should be assessed for dysfunction because this may dictate which operative side is used for the approach. If patients already have unilateral vocal cord paralysis, the same incision should be used so as not to place the contralateral vocal cord at risk. ENT should also be consulted if patients have baseline swallowing dysfunction, prior esophageal injury, or if a difficult surgical exposure is anticipated. If the soft tissue condition is in question, a plastic surgery consultation should be obtained so that complex tissue coverage is available. If patients have documented sleep apnea or pickwickian habitus, obtain a preoperative sleep study from a pulmonologist. Endocrinology can help manage osteoporosis, potentially using perioperative teriparatide (Forteo) treatment. In addition, they can optimize diabetic management to reduce the risk of wound healing problems. Rheumatology can evaluate for myopathy.

Medical photography is used to document preoperative clinical deformity and can be used as intraoperative reference. This is ideal for measuring and documenting the chin-brow vertical angle.

INDICATIONS, CONTRAINDICATIONS, AND GOALS OF SURGERY

Indications for surgery include neurologic deficit, pain, and intolerable deformity. The risk of inducing a neurologic deficit during surgery must be carefully weighed against presenting deficits and the risk of progression. Patients often find a deformity to be intolerable when it affects activities of daily living and quality of life. Deformity that causes respiratory compromise or swallowing difficulty should be corrected.

There are multiple relative contraindications to surgery. Patients with severe osteoporosis are at a higher risk of construct failure. If flap coverage is not possible over an area with poor soft tissue coverage, surgery should be avoided in that approach. Surgery should be performed in reversible dystonia only if medical management fails. Medical comorbidities may preclude lengthy, multistage procedures.

Surgical goals should be outlined with patients preoperatively to minimize unrealistic expectations. In general, the goals are to achieve a well-aligned and balanced spine, diminish pain, and correct or prevent neurologic deficits. Unfortunately, these benefits are typically counterbalanced by the loss of motion caused by a fusion. It takes a considerable amount of time to educate patients and allow them to participate in the decision making for complex cases, but that time is a good investment.

PREOPERATIVE PLANNING

Meticulous preoperative planning is necessary given the complexity of the surgery. Medical care of patients should be optimized preoperatively because their body will be in a state of catabolism postoperatively. Appropriate consultations should be obtained before surgery. If possible, chronic medical conditions should be stable and thoroughly assessed preoperatively.

When reviewing imaging, stenosis should be assessed. This condition is best seen on MRI. Stenosis can be central, foraminal, or both. The spinal cord should be assessed for myelomalacia. If stenosis is present and symptomatic, decompression should be performed. Decompression can be performed directly from the anterior. Consideration is given to the number of levels to be decompressed. Anterior multilevel corpectomies with anterior plating without supplemental posterior fixation may be associated with a high risk of complications. Indirect decompression can be performed by laminectomy or laminoplasty, allowing the spinal cord to drift posteriorly. Isolated laminoplasty or laminectomy is not recommended if patients do not have an overall neutral or lordotic cervical alignment because indirect decompression relies on the ability of the spinal cord to drift back. Surgeons should anticipate additional areas of stenosis that may develop intraoperatively after correction of the deformity.

Imaging should also be assessed for fusion. The spine can be fused congenitally, spontaneously, or surgically. Fusion can occur anteriorly, posteriorly, or circumferentially. A pseudoarthrosis is best evaluated with a CT scan and flexion/extension films. Pseudoarthrosis may be mobile or fixed and result in dynamic or static stenosis. They are often pain generators but may be asymptomatic.

Stability is assessed with flexion and extension films. Localization of instability helps guide what segments to include in fusions. Segments adjacent to deformities should be assessed for abnormal motion. Integrity of the anterior column should be assessed. If patients demonstrate rounded or wedged vertebral bodies, caution should be used when using only posterior instrumentation.

The deformity itself should be fully appreciated. Sagittal deformity is most common, but coronal deformity can occur in conjunction or isolation. Deformity should be assessed for flexibility. If a deformity is flexible, the amount of correction should be noted. Specific measurements include chin-brow to vertical angle and C1 plumb line.[14] C1 plumb line is measured with a plumb line from the tip of the odontoid in relation to the center of C7. A C7 plumb line is also measured from the center of C7 in relation to the posterior superior corner of the sacrum to assess for global imbalance in the thoracic or lumbar spine (**Fig. 4**A–G).

Special consideration should be given to patients who have had prior surgery. Prior operative reports should be obtained if possible. If planning an anterior approach on patients with previous anterior surgery, assessment of the vocal cords should be made. If paralysis on the side of previous incision is present, the contralateral side should not be used for revision surgery given the risk of complete vocal cord paralysis. Complications should be noted from previous surgeries, such as a cerebrospinal fluid (CSF) leak. Existing

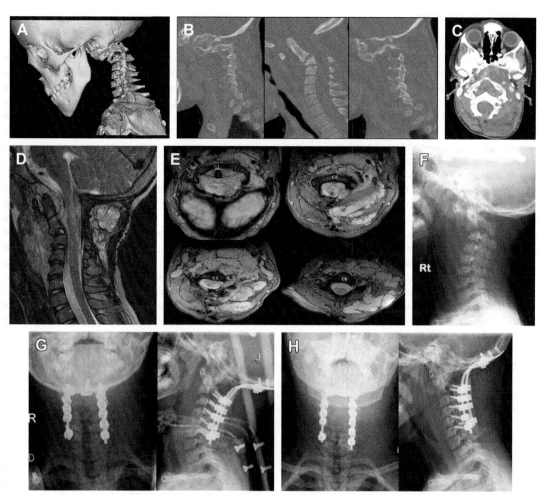

Fig. 4. A 7-year-old boy with type I neurofibromatosis. He underwent an occiput to C2 decompression in May 2007 to perform an intradural decompression of a plexiform neurofibroma that was causing myelopathy from spinal cord compression. He presented in November 2007 with progressive postlaminectomy kyphosis. His myelopathy had remained stable and he was still ambulatory with aids for his spastic gait. He was placed in halo traction for 10 days preoperatively and then underwent a single-stage posterior procedure. The intradural tumor was debulked further and the spine was fused with a rod/screw construct from occiput to C6 using BMP-2, MasterGraft (Medtronic, Minneapolis, Minnesota; off label) and iliac crest autograft. He was immobilized in a halo vest postoperatively for 3 months. Open reduction was achieved indirectly at the time of surgery through manipulation of the halo and directly by pressing anteriorly on C3 while translating the occiput posteriorly. The rods were compressed between C2 and 3 to reduce that level further after removing the facet capsules and cartilage from the facet joints. The authors did not expose the lateral masses of C1, rather C1 moved with the occiput and was reduced relative to C2 during the translation maneuver. The authors were prepared to do a subsequent anterior fusion if the posterior fusion did not heal or he started to loose correction but that was not necessary. He will need to be followed for life because of the likely tumor regrowth. (*A*) A 3-dimensional CT reformatted image demonstrating deformity. (*B*) CT sagittal reformatted images (*left, center, right*). He has cranial settling with the tip of the odontoid inside the foramen magnum. C1 is dislocated anteriorly relative to C2 on the right and markedly subluxed on the left. C2 has subluxed anteriorly relative to C3. The posterior elements are deficient from prior suboccipital craniotomy and laminectomies of C1 and C2. The C3 vertebral body is compressed anteriorly, and he has a severe postlaminectomy kyphotic deformity from C2 to 4. (*C*) Axial CT demonstrating the C1-2 dislocation. (*D*) Sagittal T2-weighted MRI from September 2007 demonstrating extensive plexiform neurofibroma involving intradural and extradural spaces C1-2 as well as the extraspinal soft tissues posteriorly and the retropharyngeal space. The progressive nature of the deformity can be appreciated by comparing this image with the reformatted CT in Fig. 4(*B*) taken just 2 months later. (*E*) Axial T2-weighted MRI images from September 2007 demonstrating extensive tumor involvement throughout the neck. (*F*) Lateral radiograph after 1 week in 4.5 kg of traction showing partial reduction of the deformity. Traction was begun with just 1.8 kg of weight and close observation. (*G*) Anteroposterior and lateral radiographs taken with the patient in a halo during the immediate postoperative period. (*H*) Anteroposterior and lateral radiographs taken nearly 3 years postoperatively showing solid posterior fusion, no loss of alignment, and remodeling of the C3 vertebral body. He had not had any additional surgery. His neurologic status is stable, he has no pain, and he is still ambulatory.

implants should be identified on operative reports or, if possible, on imaging. Instrumentation specific to the system in place should be on hand to help with removal. Otherwise, a universal removal set or metal cutting burr should be available. If a prior laminectomy was performed, its extent should be noted to try and decrease the chance of CSF leak or cord injury during exposure. Wide laminectomy makes the spine less stable and will more likely require anterior-posterior fusion.

Imaging should be used to assess degeneration of adjacent joints. The planned construct should be extended to include adjacent degenerated joints to prevent junctional breakdown.

In upper cervical fusions, contrast imaging should be used to assess the course and dominance of the vertebral arteries and the location of the internal carotid arteries relative to the anterior arch of the atlas. In the subaxial spine, the anatomy of the vertebral arteries can be assessed with plain CT and MRI scans. Congenital bony anomalies should be noted in addition to vascular anomalies.

Soft tissue assessment is vital. If there is contracture or poor integrity of the soft tissues, patients may require soft tissue flap coverage postoperatively. If the anterior tissues have been contracted for an extended period of time, patients may develop difficulty swallowing postoperatively and require a percutaneous feeding tube for nutrition. If the posterior musculature is poor from myopathy or extensive radiation therapy, the posterior construct will likely need to be extended to C2.

SELECTION OF LEVELS

The extent of the instrumentation and fusion should be decided based on multiple factors. The cause, location, type of prior surgery (if any), and quality of bone are all factored into the decision.[2,15] In general, the most cephalad and caudal vertebral bodies involved in the deformity curve are the beginning and end of the extent of the fusion. However, if the posterior musculature is weak, the bone is severely osteoporotic, or the cause is metastatic disease, the fusion should be extended longer, often to C2. Posteriorly, C2 offers a stronger point of fixation compared with C3 and allows for improved correction and stabilization. The C7 lateral mass is often difficult to instrument because of its size; a pedicle screw can be used at this level. The position of a C7 pedicle screw can be challenging to connect to a C6 lateral mass screw. In addition, stopping a construct at C7 is often avoided because of the concentration of stress at the cervicothoracic junction. For these reasons, C2 and T2 are common endpoints on posterior constructs, with C7 sometimes remaining uninstrumented.[4] If a prior laminectomy has been performed, the length of the laminectomy should be fused, plus one normal vertebrae above and below the fusion segment.

STAGING

Determination of the number and sequence of stages of surgery should be planned. Isolated anterior surgery is an option provided that there is not a fusion posteriorly or ankylosis of the facet joints. In addition, the construct itself should be short because the risk of pseudoarthrosis increases with longer anterior constructs.

Posterior procedures can be performed in isolation with specific indications. The deformity can be a flexible kyphosis with an unfused anterior column. Posterior procedures can also be performed when kyphosis is caused by ankylosing spondylitis.[2] Kyphosis in the setting of rounded vertebral bodies indicates that the anterior column has lost its integrity and an isolated posterior fusion may fail.

Two-stage combined procedures, also referred to as 360° reconstructions, are indicated when stability needs to be augmented. Instability may be caused by prior laminectomy, adjacent level disease in a previous 360° reconstruction, trauma with significant ligamentous injury, or multilevel corpectomies. A 360° reconstruction should also be considered in patients who are at significant risk for developing a pseudoarthrosis, such as a smoker with anterior cervical discectomy and fusion at 3 or more levels.[16] The addition of the posterior approach also allows for dorsal decompression of the spinal cord, if necessary.[2] A 360° reconstruction permits immediate rigid stabilization and eliminates the need for halo immobilization postoperatively. Higher rates of fusion have been demonstrated with the combined approach compared with the isolated anterior approach.[17] Correction of deformity with a 360° reconstruction is typically possible when only the anterior or posterior aspect of the spine is fused.

If both the anterior and posterior aspects of the spine are fused, a 3-stage combined procedure (540°) is usually required. This procedure allows for osteotomies to be performed anteriorly and posteriorly. In general, the first stage serves as a release osteotomy with partial correction. The second stage completes the correction and provides some fixation. The third stage augments the fixation across initial releases. Wollowick and colleagues[18] reported performing anterior osteotomies that partially correct the deformity through plastic deformation through a weak posterior fusion followed by further deformity correction via posterior osteotomies and fusion. The authors prefer a 3-stage procedure for more control and less risk of anterior vertebral body disruption caused by forceful manipulation of the spine with distracting devices. Three-stage procedures are also indicated when prior posterior instrumentation is in place and requires removal before anterior correction. All 3 stages are not done on the same day because of the length of surgical time required. In general, the first stage can be done on the first day. The second and third stages are done on a second day because the third stage normally involves placing instrumentation and is relatively quick.

PREOPERATIVE TRACTION

The need for preoperative traction should be determined. Traction can be used to gradually straighten an unfused but stiff deformity. In addition, it allows us to monitor neurologic status during correction, which is especially helpful in cases whereby it is unclear if a single approach would be adequate or in cases whereby neurologic status is tenuous. If reduction is significant after a few days in traction, a posterior instrumentation and fusion can be used to maintain the correction. If there is no correction with traction over a few days, it is unlikely that traction will provide correction, and a 360° approach is necessary. Preoperative traction should be used sparingly. Patient compliance can be an issue. Complications of transient neurologic deterioration and medical complications have been reported.[19] In addition, patients must remain in the hospital preoperatively, placing them at higher risk of a nosocomial infection (**Fig. 5A–H**).

OSTEOTOMIES

The location, type, and magnitude of osteotomies to be performed should be determined. Smith-Peterson osteotomies of the spine were first described in 1945.[20] Use of osteotomy in the cervical spine was reported by Mason and colleagues.[21] Simmons[22] was the first to publish a series of corrective osteotomies at the cervicothoracic junction.

The Smith-Peterson osteotomy involves the resection of posterior elements through the facet joints and pars intra-articularis. Laminectomies are performed at C6, C7, and T1. The C8 nerve roots are widely decompressed. The posterior column is closed, and the anterior column opens through the disk space. All 3 columns are disrupted, rendering the spine unstable until it is reconstructed.[18]

Pedicle subtraction osteotomy (PSO) is indicated in large deformities, especially those that are sharp and angular. It involves a closing wedge osteotomy that hinges on the anterior longitudinal ligament and anterior aspect of the vertebral body. Bilateral lamina and facets are resected. The pedicles and vertebral body are decancellated. The posterior vertebral cortex is collapsed into the decancellated vertebral body defect, and the lateral cortex is resected. The osteotomy site is closed, creating bony apposition of the vertebral body and posterior elements. An asymmetric osteotomy can be done to correct a coexistent coronal deformity.[23] Greater blood loss occurs with PSO, but greater correction is obtained. The correction obtained in a PSO is comparable with that obtained with 3 Smith-Peterson osteotomies.[24]

Osteotomies are performed in the region of maximal deformity while also taking into account possible complications. The cervicothoracic junction is most commonly chosen because of the large size of the spinal canal at this level, safety in relation to the location of the vertebral artery, and the mobility of the spinal cord and C8 nerve roots. In the event of a C8 nerve injury, most hand function is still possible.[18]

ANESTHESIA AND POSITIONING

Surgical correction of complex deformity can be performed with patients under local anesthesia and conscious sedation in a sitting position. This practice allows for an easier wake-up test and gradual, controlled correction of deformity.[25] However, neurologic deficits, including quadriplegia, have been reported even when surgery is performed in this position.[26]

General anesthesia with monitoring can be used. Langeloo and colleagues[27] studied 16 patients who underwent C7 osteotomy with internal fixation. Eleven patients were in a sitting position and 5 were prone. Longer fusion constructs down to T4–T6 were able to be done in the prone group, allowing them to be immobilized in a cervical orthosis postoperatively. The sitting group required halo-cast immobilization postoperatively. All patients achieved union without loss of correction.

The authors prefer to use general anesthesia with patients in the prone position and multimodality intraoperative monitoring (IOM). Intravenous anesthetic is used because of the interference of gas anesthesia with IOM. In a recent report, 102 consecutive adults underwent IOM during corrective surgery for spinal deformity, and the accuracy of IOM was compared with postoperative examination. Multimodality IOM via somatosensory-evoked potentials (SEPs), motor-evoked potentials (MEPs), and EMG were found to have an overall sensitivity of 100% and specificity of 84.3%. Sensitivity was 67% and specificity was 98% in patients undergoing major deformity correction. The investigators concluded that IOM allowed for the early detection of neural injury that allowed them to restore blood pressure and avoid overcorrection or forgo the osteotomy to try and avoid postoperative paraparesis.[28] In 2010, Fehlings and colleagues[29] performed a meta-analysis of IOM. They found that multimodality intraoperative neuromonitoring is sensitive

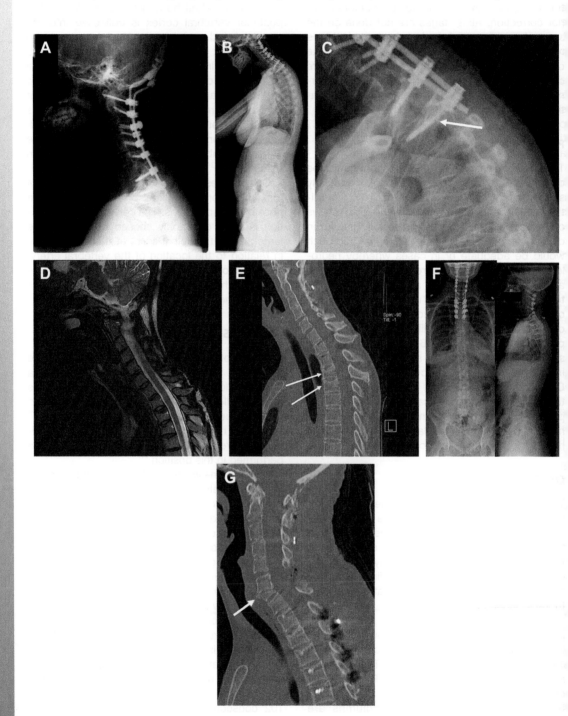

and specific for detecting intraoperative neurologic injury and should be considered during deformity correction and instrumentation. The authors prefer anesthesia to maintain mean arterial pressures (MAPs) more than 80 mmHg throughout the procedure and increase it to 90 mm Hg at the time of osteotomy closure. In addition, if IOM demonstrates an amplitude loss of at least 60% and is sustained for more than 10 minutes, MAPs are increased to 90 mm HG.[30] If there continues to be concern regarding IOM, a wake-up test is performed.

When performing posterior osteotomies, the authors prefer to use the prone position. A Jackson frame (Mizuho OSI, Union City, CA, USA) is set up with a chest bolster, anterior iliac crest pads, anterior thigh pads, and a leg sling. Additional padding or pillows may be necessary to accommodate thoracic or thoracolumbar deformity. The authors prefer the use of a Mayfield head clamp (Ohio Medical Instrument Co., Cincinatti, OH, USA) with pinions because of its stability. Other authors prefer securing the head with Gardner-Wells tongs with 6.8 kg of weight in bivector traction. If bivector traction is used, one rope should be in line with deformity and the other rope directs the head into extension.[18]

Once patients are in the prone positione, it is important to assess the position of the spine clinically. The chin-brow to Jackson table angle should be noted and compared with the goal correction angle. The coronal and axial alignment is best checked by looking at the patients' head position from underneath the operating table. The table is placed in the reverse Trendelenburg position to decrease facial swelling and to attempt to make the surgical field level for surgeon comfort.

SPINAL NAVIGATION

The authors prefer to use spinal navigation during complex deformity correction. In a recent systematic review and meta-analysis, the use of navigation allowed more accurate pedicle screw placement than conventional techniques and the accuracy was even greater for deformity cases.[31] The benefit of navigation is a possible improvement in safety and accuracy. This navigation is

---

Fig. 5. A 27-year-old woman with juvenile RA presented in January 2008 with complaints of right occipital pain for 5 years and bilateral radicular symptoms for 6 months. She was found to have spontaneous fusions occiput to C1 and C2-C5, marked destruction of the right C1-2 joint with minimal basilar invagination. She had foraminal stenosis at C5-6 and C6-7. She underwent occiput to T2 posterior instrumented spinal fusion with bilateral C5-6 and left C6-7 foraminotomies. She did well initially with resolution of occipital neuralgia and radiculopathy. She developed upper thoracic pain and progressive flexion deformity of her neck and was found to have developed compression fractures of T3 and T4 and fractures of the T2 pedicle screws. She underwent a C7 pedicle subtraction osteotomy and fusion with reinstrumentation C1 to T6 with iliac crest and local bone graft. Intraoperative image guidance, multimodality neural monitoring, and an operating microscope were used. No changes were detected with the SEPs or MEPs, and there were no neurotonic discharges on free-running EMG. However, the patient awoke with partial left C7 and C8 palsies. CT and MRI did not reveal any significant problems, but the foramen on the left that now contained both the C7 and C8 roots was snug. She was given intravenous steroids and observed initially, but after several days she elected to undergo another procedure to widen the foramen. The authors partially opened the osteotomy site and inspected neural elements. They found that the C7 and C8 roots were touching and there was a minor degree of foraminal stenosis, which was decompressed. The dura was kinking on closing the osteotomy site, but an intraoperative ultrasound revealed good CSF flow around the cord and no stenosis. The instrumentation was reinserted and the patient made an uneventful recovery. Her palsies had markedly improved after 2 months. At her 1-year follow-up, her palsies were almost completely resolved, she had rhomboid discomfort but was more functional and was pleased with her head alignment. (A) Standing lateral cervical radiograph after her index occiput-T2 fusion operation. Her chin-brow-vertical angle was 10°, as she had requested preoperatively. (B) Long-standing spine radiographs 1.5 years following her index procedure and before the PSO show that the C7 plumb line falls just at the back of the L5-S1 disk. In this position, her chin-brow-vertical angle measures 39°. (C) Enlarged view from Fig. 5(A) showing the broken screws at T2 (arrow) and compression fractures at T3 and T4. (D) Sagittal T2-weighted MRI before the PSO shows no stenosis but she has compression fractures of T3 and 4. Her bone mineral density was normal (T-score was 0.3 at the hip and -0.5 L at spine). (E) CT sagittal reformatted image demonstrates same findings as MRI in Fig. 5(D), compression fractures T3 and 4 (arrows). No pseudoarthrosis was seen on the lateral images despite the broken screws at T2. (F) Final long-standing posteroanterior and lateral radiographs show excellent alignment with chin-brow-vertical angle 0°. The authors normally strive to place the neck in slight flexion because it is thought to be a more functional alignment, but the patient requested that they make the chin-brow-vertical angle neutral because she thought that the initial 10° achieved at the first operation was too flexed. The broken screws were left in the vertebral bodies of T2. (G) Final postoperative sagittal reformatted CT demonstrating the PSO at C7. There is a small fracture on the anterior aspect of the C7 vertebral body (arrow). Ideally, the osteotomy would not involve the anterior wall of the vertebral body to avoid instability with translation.

most helpful when the spine is already fused from prior surgery or AS and the landmarks are distorted. Navigation is also helpful in patients with small pedicles and bony anomalies. The disadvantage is increased operative time and added expense to a surgery that is already lengthy and costly. In addition, there is always the possibility of registration error that could give the surgeon a false sense of security.

SURGICAL TECHNIQUE

In anterior cases, a standard Smith-Robinson approach is used with patients on a radiolucent table. If patients have had prior anterior surgery and preoperative work-up identified that the vocal cord has normal function on the side of the incision, the contralateral side is used for the approach to avoid scar tissue and provide an easier dissection. If the vocal cord has lost function on the side of the incision, the same incision should be used so as not to risk complete paralysis of the vocal cords.

In posterior cases, a midline incision is used. Subperiosteal dissection is performed to the lateral border of the lateral masses. Additional dissection laterally will lead to unnecessary bleeding. Meticulous hemostasis is maintained to minimize blood loss. Care is taken not to disrupt facet joints that are not to be included in the fusion. After exposure, an intraoperative CT scan may be obtained for use with navigation, if available. Pedicle screws are typically placed at C7 and in the thoracic spine, and lateral mass screws are placed from C3 to C6. If extending up to C2, the authors prefer to use pars screws; however, pedicle screws or laminar screws can also be used.

If an osteotomy is required, a temporary rod is used to provisionally hold the spine secure during the osteotomy and to prevent inadvertent translation. This rod is made by contouring a malleable rod template to fit into the screws before osteotomy. A titanium rod is bent to match the rod template and is provisionally secured to the screws. A second rod is bent similarly and then further contoured to conform to the planned corrective bend at the osteotomy site. The second rod replaces the first one at the time of osteotomy closure. Alternatively, commercially available hinged rods can be used for this purpose.

Cervical extension osteotomies are most commonly performed at C7. A complete laminectomy of C7 is performed with a high-speed bur. If the lamina and spinous process can be removed as a single unit, it should be saved for bone graft. Bone removed with Kerrison rongeurs can also be saved for bone graft. The inferior half of the C6 lamina and the superior half of the T1 lamina are removed. The facets and lateral masses of C7 are removed. The caudal aspect of the inferior facet of C6 and the cranial aspect of the superior facet of T1 should be excised. The C7 and C8 nerve roots are visualized and protected. The C7 pedicles and vertebral body are decancellated with a bur and curettes. The remaining C7 pedicle walls are resected. A Woodson elevator or reversed curette is placed in front of the posterior longitudinal ligament and used to push through the dorsal cortex into the cavity created in the C7 vertebral body. The first temporary rod is removed and the precontoured rod is connected to the thoracic pedicle screws. The MAP is increased to 90 mm, and an unscrubbed assistant unlocks the Mayfield and extends the neck. If bivector traction is used instead of the Mayfield device, the traction weight is switched to the extension rope at this point. The Mayfield is locked into position with the surgeon watching the spine and the unscrubbed assistant assessing the postcorrected chin-brow to table angle and coronal and axial alignment. The spinal cord, C7, and C8 nerve roots should be visualized to ensure that adequate bone was resected to prevent postoperative central or foraminal stenosis. The rod is seated in the proximal screws, and the opposite-side rod is contoured and secured to the spine. Multimodal IOM is checked throughout the procedure. If there are significant changes in latency or amplitude on the SEPs or MEPs or neurotonic discharges on the free running EMG monitoring, the MAP is elevated, the rods are released proximally, correction is reduced, and the decompression site is inspected. Further decompression is performed as needed. Images should be obtained to determine if translation has occurred. A wake-up test may be required. Assuming the IOM returns to baseline, the correction maneuver may be repeated. If the IOM does not return to baseline, it may be necessary to temporarily secure the spine in the uncorrected position and abort the procedure to assess the patients' neurologic status and perform further imaging.

Once the osteotomy site is closed, the spine is stabilized with the rods and cross-links are added, if deemed necessary. The wound is thoroughly irrigated. Local autograft is used as bone graft and augmented as needed. Typically, one drain is placed deep to the fascia and another is placed superficial to the fascia (see **Fig. 5D–F**).

POSTOPERATIVE MANAGEMENT

If patients are undergoing staged procedures, they may be kept intubated for airway protection between stages. Regarding extubation, a cuff-leak test should be performed before extubation, and patients may remain intubated overnight. Risk factors for delayed extubation include extended operative time greater than 10 hours, obesity, transfusion of greater than 3 to 4 units of blood, 4-level anterior surgery, and revision anterior surgery.[32,33]

Immobilization type and duration are based on stability and bone quality. Variation exists with surgeon preference. Most patients are immobilized in a soft or hard cervical collar for 6 to 12 weeks. Occasionally, immobilization is extended up with a halo or down with a cervicothoracic orthosis if fusion includes C2 or the cervicothoracic junction, respectively.[34]

Patients are encouraged to ambulate. Their pain is initially controlled with patient-controlled intravenous analgesia until they demonstrate the ability to swallow. If they have difficulty swallowing, a swallowing study is obtained to avoid aspiration.

ADDITIONAL PEARLS

Preoperative planning is the key to success. It is important to incorporate contingency options into the preoperative plan, and these should be discussed with patients. Considerable time should be spent with patients preoperatively so they have realistic expectations and a firm understanding of the high-risk nature of cervical deformity surgery. Additional surgical stages may be required if adequate correction is not achieved, stability is questionable, or delayed union occurs. The fusion construct may need to be extended intraoperatively. If additional points of fixation are needed. Additional decompression may be required if IOM suggests a problem. Different fixation options should be planned in case fixation points are inadequate. For example, if fixation is to include C2, intralaminar screws can be used if pedicle or pars screws are not possible or have poor fixation. Finally, postoperative debriefing and good communication are essential. If multidisciplinary teams are involved, clarification should be given about the type of suction to be used on drains, dressings, and activities because common practice in some disciplines can be deleterious in specific circumstances. For example, placing a drain to wall suction in the setting of an unrecognized CSF leak can exacerbate the leak.

SUMMARY

Complex spinal deformities can be debilitating for patients, affecting quality of life. It is important to understand the cause, clinical manifestations, and the patients' goals because these factors may impact treatment options. Multiple techniques exist, and surgical treatment should be individualized. Regardless of the approach chosen, careful preoperative planning and meticulous surgical technique are essential.

REFERENCES

1. Basu PS, Elsebaie H, Noordeen MH. Congenital spinal deformity: a comprehensive assessment at presentation. Spine (Phila Pa 1976) 2002;27:2255–9.
2. Han K, Lu C, Li J, et al. Surgical treatment of cervical kyphosis. Eur Spine J 2011;20:523–36.
3. Chi JH, Tay B, Stahl D, et al. Complex deformities of the cervical spine. Neurosurg Clin N Am 2007;18: 295–304.
4. Hiratzka J. Degenerative cervical kyphosis: treatment, complications, and outcomes. Semin Spine Surg 2011;23:165–9.
5. Barsa P, Suchomel P. Factors affecting sagittal malalignment due to cage subsidence in standalone cage assisted anterior cervical fusion. Eur Spine J 2007;16:1395–400.
6. Rhee JM. Iatrogenic cervical deformity. Semin Spine Surg 2011;23:173–80.
7. Wang JC, McDonough PW, Endow K, et al. The effect of cervical plating on single-level anterior cervical discectomy and fusion. J Spinal Disord 1999;12:467–71.
8. Wang JC, McDonough PW, Endow KK, et al. Increased fusion rates with cervical plating for two-level anterior cervical discectomy and fusion. Spine (Phila Pa 1976) 2000;25:41–5.
9. Kaptain GJ, Simmons NE, Replogle RE, et al. Incidence and outcome of kyphotic deformity following laminectomy for cervical spondylotic myelopathy. J Neurosurg 2000;93:199–204.
10. Suk KS, Kim KT, Lee JH, et al. Sagittal alignment of the cervical spine after the laminoplasty. Spine (Phila Pa 1976) 2007;32:E656–60.
11. Hohl JB, Grabowski G, Donaldson WF. Cervical deformity in rheumatoid arthritis. Semin Spine Surg 2011;23:181–7.
12. Gerling MC, Bohlman HH. Dropped head deformity due to cervical myopathy: surgical treatment outcomes and complications spanning twenty years. Spine 2008;33:E739–45.
13. Suk KS, Kim KT, Lee SH, et al. Significance of chin-brow vertical angle in correction of kyphotic deformity of ankylosing spondylitis patients. Spine (Phila Pa 1976) 2003;28:2001–5.
14. Hardacker JW, Shuford RF, Capicotto PN, et al. Radiographic standing cervical segmental alignment in adult volunteers without neck symptoms. Spine (Phila Pa 1976) 1997;22:1472–80 [discussion: 1480].

15. Steinmetz MP, Kager CD, Benzel EC. Ventral correction of postsurgical cervical kyphosis. J Neurosurg 2003;98:1–7.

16. Nottmeier EW, Deen HG, Patel N, et al. Cervical kyphotic deformity correction using 360-degree reconstruction. J Spinal Disord Tech 2009;22:385–91.

17. Schultz KD Jr, McLaughlin MR, Haid RW Jr, et al. Single-stage anterior-posterior decompression and stabilization for complex cervical spine disorders. J Neurosurg 2000;93:214–21.

18. Wollowick AL, Kelly MP, Riew KD. Osteotomies for the treatment of cervical kyphosis caused by ankylosing spondylitis: indications and techniques. Semin Spine Surg 2011;23:188–98.

19. Herman JM, Sonntag VK. Cervical corpectomy and plate fixation for postlaminectomy kyphosis. J Neurosurg 1994;80:963–70.

20. Smith-Petersen MN, Larson CB, Aufranc OE. Osteotomy of the spine for correction of flexion deformity in rheumatoid arthritis. Clin Orthop Relat Res 1969;66:6–9.

21. Mason C, Cozen L, Adelstein L. Surgical correction of flexion deformity of the cervical spine. Calif Med 1953;79:244–6.

22. Simmons EH. The surgical correction of flexion deformity of the cervical spine in ankylosing spondylitis. Clin Orthop Relat Res 1972;86:132–43.

23. Mummaneni PV, Mummaneni VP, Haid RW Jr, et al. Cervical osteotomy for the correction of chin-on-chest deformity in ankylosing spondylitis. Technical note. Neurosurg Focus 2003;14:e9.

24. Cho KJ, Bridwell KH, Lenke LG, et al. Comparison of Smith-Petersen versus pedicle subtraction osteotomy for the correction of fixed sagittal imbalance. Spine (Phila Pa 1976) 2005;30:2030–7 [discussion: 2038].

25. Bouchard JA, Feibel RJ. Gradual multiplanar cervical osteotomy to correct kyphotic ankylosing spondylitic deformities. Can J Surg 2002;45:215–8.

26. Belanger TA, Milam RA 4th, Roh JS, et al. Cervicothoracic extension osteotomy for chin-on-chest deformity in ankylosing spondylitis. J Bone Joint Surg Am 2005;87:1732–8.

27. Langeloo DD, Journee HL, Pavlov PW, et al. Cervical osteotomy in ankylosing spondylitis: evaluation of new developments. Eur Spine J 2006;15:493–500.

28. Quraishi NA, Lewis SJ, Kelleher MO, et al. Intraoperative multimodality monitoring in adult spinal deformity: analysis of a prospective series of one hundred two cases with independent evaluation. Spine (Phila Pa 1976) 2009;34:1504–12.

29. Fehlings MG, Brodke DS, Norvell DC, et al. The evidence for intraoperative neurophysiological monitoring in spine surgery: does it make a difference? Spine (Phila Pa 1976) 2010;35:S37–46.

30. Hilibrand AS, Schwartz DM, Sethuraman V, et al. Comparison of transcranial electric motor and somatosensory evoked potential monitoring during cervical spine surgery. J Bone Joint Surg Am 2004;86:1248–53.

31. Tian NF, Huang QS, Zhou P, et al. Pedicle screw insertion accuracy with different assisted methods: a systematic review and meta-analysis of comparative studies. Eur Spine J 2011;20:846–59.

32. Kwon B, Yoo JU, Furey CG, et al. Risk factors for delayed extubation after single-stage, multi-level anterior cervical decompression and posterior fusion. J Spinal Disord Tech 2006;19:389–93.

33. Epstein NE, Hollingsworth R, Nardi D, et al. Can airway complications following multilevel anterior cervical surgery be avoided? J Neurosurg 2001;94:185–8.

34. Mummaneni PV, Dhall SS, Rodts GE, et al. Circumferential fusion for cervical kyphotic deformity. J Neurosurg Spine 2008;9:515–21.

Revision Cervical Spine Surgery

Jeffrey A. Rihn, MD*, Chambliss Harrod, MD,
Todd J. Albert, MD

KEYWORDS

- Revision surgery • Cervical spine
- Adjacent segment disease • Same segment disease

Revision cervical spine surgery can be a complex and risky endeavor. The indications for revision surgery are numerous and include pseudarthrosis, infection, adjacent segment disease, same segment disease, instrumentation failure, and progressive deformity. The evaluation, diagnosis, and management of each of these problems can be challenging. It is essential that the underlying problem be identified through a comprehensive history taking and physical examination as well as appropriate imaging studies. It is also essential to understand why the initial procedure failed so that a similar situation can be avoided during revision surgery. When planning revision surgery, the surgeon must consider the cause of the underlying problem (eg, biological, mechanical, and so forth), the potential for complications, and clinical outcomes that can reasonably be expected. This information should be clearly explained to the patient during the informed consent process. This article provides the spine care provider with an understanding of how to appropriately evaluate and manage the most common cervical conditions that require revision cervical spine surgery.

CONSIDERATIONS FOR REVISION SURGERY
History Taking

Patient history and examination are essential to determining whether or not a patient is a candidate for revision cervical spine surgery. History taking should include a thorough discussion of the initial procedure. Questions that should be asked include the following: why did you have your initial procedure; what symptoms were you having before your initial procedure; following the initial procedure, did you get relief from some or all of your symptoms; if so, how long did this relief last; are the symptoms you are having now similar to those you had before your initial procedure; and if not, how are the symptoms different. These questions will give the spine care provider some sense of whether the initial problem was successfully treated and whether the current symptoms represent persistence of the initial problem, recurrence of the initial problem, or a new problem at an adjacent level. Questions regarding constitutional symptoms (ie, fever, chills, nausea, vomiting, unexplained weight loss, fatigue) should also be addressed during the history taking to assess for problems such as infection or tumor. Questions pertinent to the nature, duration, severity, and location of pain, numbness, and/or tingling as well as questions relating to weakness, problems with balance and fine motor skills, and bowel and bladder function are essential as they are when assessing any spine patient. Red flags such as progressive weakness, constitutional symptoms, and unrelenting pain are suggestive of an urgent or even emergent situation. The patient should also be asked about hoarseness and/or swallowing problems that may be attributed to the initial procedure and may affect the surgical approach for the current problem.

Physical Examination

Whether a patient presents for primary or recurrent problem, a thorough physical examination is indicated that includes inspection, palpation, range of motion test, a full neurologic evaluation, and

Department of Orthopaedic Surgery, Thomas Jefferson University and Hospitals, The Rothman Institute, 925 Chestnut Street, 5th floor, Philadelphia, PA 19107, USA
* Corresponding author. Thomas Jefferson University Hospital, The Rothman Institute, 925 Chestnut Street, 5th Floor, Philadelphia, PA 19107.
E-mail address: jrihno16@yahoo.com

Orthop Clin N Am 43 (2012) 123–136
doi:10.1016/j.ocl.2011.09.001
0030-5898/12/$ – see front matter © 2012 Published by Elsevier Inc

orthopedic.theclinics.com

provocative tests specific to the cervical spine. It is not uncommon that shoulder, elbow, or wrist pathology can mimic cervical spine pathology. Such pathologic conditions must be ruled out during the patient evaluation to avoid unnecessary revision cervical spine surgery. This is particularly true when the initial procedure did not provide any relief of the patient's original symptoms, suggesting that pathologic condition of the upper extremity rather than the cervical may be the cause of the original symptoms. On inspection, the location and appearance of the initial incision should be noted. Erythema, incisional drainage, and incisional tenderness may indicate the presence of infection. The side of the incision is particularly important when performing anterior cervical surgery because it oftentimes dictates the side of the approach during revision surgery.

Imaging

Imaging techniques that are most often used to evaluate a patient for revision cervical spine surgery include plain radiography, computed tomographic (CT) scan, and magnetic resonance imaging (MRI). Plain radiography should typically include anteroposterior, lateral, and flexion/extension views. Cervical alignment (ie, loss of lordosis, kyphosis) should be measured on the lateral radiograph. The status of an existing fusion should be assessed, looking for the presence of bridging trabecular bone or continued motion. The presence and location of instrumentation should be noted. Subtle loosing of existing screws in the form of haloing can indicate pseudarthrosis (Fig. 1). Implant failure in the form of screw pullout and screw and/or rod breakage should be noted.

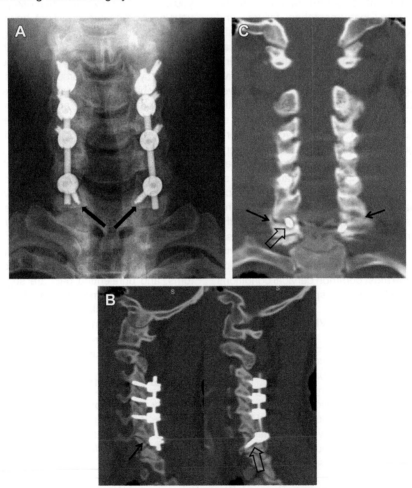

Fig. 1. (A) Postoperative anteroposterior cervical radiograph of a patient 12 months after a posterior cervical laminectomy and fusion from C3 to C7. Haloing is seen around the bilateral C7 pedicle screws (black arrows). (B) Postoperative sagittal CT reconstructions of the cervical spine at the same follow-up, again demonstrating haloing (open black arrow, right). The CT demonstrates a solid bony fusion from C3 to C6 but a pseudarthrosis at C6-7 (solid black arrow, left). (C) Postoperative coronal CT reconstruction also demonstrates the solid fusion from C3 to C6, the pseudarthrosis at C6-7 (solid black arrows), and haloing (open black arrow).

Catastrophic failure of implants can be seen in the setting of spinal instability (ie, from trauma, tumor, or infection) or deformity treated with an instrumentation construct that provides inadequate biomechanical stabilization. Infection and pseudarthrosis should also be considered when subtle or overt signs of instrumentation loosening or failure are noted on radiographs. Flexion and extension lateral cervical radiographs are helpful in assessing for pseudarthrosis and instability. Excessive motion (ie, >2-mm difference, measured between the spinous processes on flexion and extension radiographs) suggests that the fusion, often an anterior cervical diskectomy and fusion (ACDF), is not fully healed. Flexion and extension radiographs may also show movement of loosening screws and angular motion that also suggests pseudarthrosis and/or instability (**Fig. 2**). Instrumented posterior cervical fusions that develop pseudarthrosis may not move on flexion and extension but may rather show screw breakage or loosening.

CT scan is helpful in identifying uncovertebral osteophytes and neuroforaminal narrowing in the setting of same segment or adjacent segment disease. CT scan is commonly used as the imaging modality of choice to assess patients with previous cervical fusion and possible pseudarthrosis. Coronal and sagittal reconstructions are particularly helpful in assessing the fusion as well as the position and status of the instrumentation. Anterior cervical fusion after corpectomy and/or diskectomy and posterior cervical fusion between the lateral masses and facet joints can be assessed with great detail using CT scan. Bridging trabecular bone in these areas indicate a solid fusion. Lucency that is typically linear in nature indicates a pseudarthrosis. Lytic bony destruction may be seen in cases of infection or tumor. Loosening of the instrumentation in the form of haloing and/or overt screw pullout can be noted. Screw and rod breakage may or may not be noted on CT scan and, in many cases, is better assessed during plain radiography (ie, static and

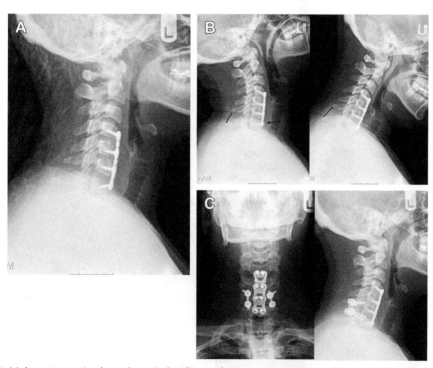

Fig. 2. (*A*) Initial postoperative lateral cervical radiographs in a patient who underwent an anterior cervical discectomy and fusion from C4 to C7, demonstrating acceptable position of the bone grafts and instrumentation. (*B*) Flexion (*right*) and extension (*left*) lateral cervical radiographs obtained 10 months postoperatively demonstrate a solid fusion at C4-5 and C5-6 but persistent motion when comparing both the radiographs between the C6 and C7 spinous processes (*black lines*) that measured 2.5 mm. In addition to the persistent motion, one of the C7 screws has loosened and backed out (*black arrow*). These findings are consistent with a pseudarthrosis at C6-7. (*C*) Anteroposterior (*left*) and lateral (*right*) cervical radiographs taken after the patient was taken back to the operating room for posterior cervical instrumentation and fusion at C6-7 with C6 lateral mass screws and C7 pedicle screws.

dynamic studies) (**Fig. 3**). CT scan can also show in detail bony destruction because of loose instrumentation, infection, and/or tumor. The status of the bone should be noted, particularly if revision instrumentation is planned. Significant bony destruction precludes the placement of instrumentation and can alter the surgical plan, oftentimes leading to proximal and/or distal extension of the instrumentation into areas of preserved bony anatomy.

MRI provides great detail of the soft tissue structures of the cervical spine, including the intervertebral disk, interspinous ligaments, and neural structures. It is used to aid in the diagnosis of same segment and adjacent segment disease, spinal cord compression, infection, and tumor. Postoperatively, MRI is helpful in identifying deep epidural fluid collections that can represent infection. In patients who have had prior cervical surgery, MRI of the cervical spine can be performed with and without gadolinium. This helps differentiate recurrent disease and/or fluid collections from scar tissue. Scar tissue is vascular and therefore enhances after the intravenous administration of gadolinium, which has a high signal intensity on the T1-weighted image. Herniated intervertebral disks and fluid collections; however, are avascular and generally have a low signal intensity on the T1-weighted image. In patients who cannot have an MRI, CT myelography is helpful when assessing the neurologic structures for evidence of compression.

Additional Testing

Certain laboratory tests can be helpful in working up a patient for revision cervical spine surgery. If there is a concern that the patient may have an

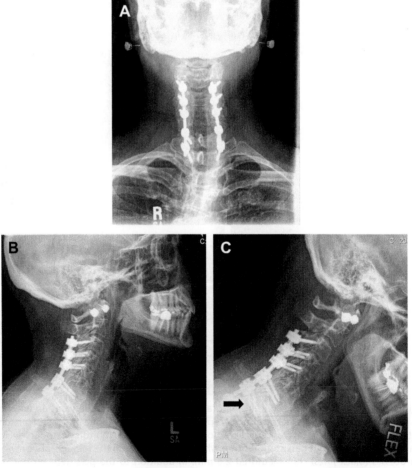

Fig. 3. (A) Anteroposterior and (B) lateral cervical radiographs in a patient 16 months after a posterior cervical laminectomy and fusion from C3 to T1 with increased neck pain over the last 4 weeks. These radiographs do not show any evidence of instrumentation failure. (C) A flexion lateral cervical radiograph, however, shows that both T1 screws are broken (*black arrow*), suggesting an underlying pseudarthrosis.

infection, a complete white blood cell count with differentiation, an erythrocyte sedimentation rate (ESR), and determination of C-reactive protein (CRP) level should be recommended. Elevation of 1 or all of these markers should raise suspicion of infection. ESR and CRP are both nonspecific markers of inflammation. CRP is a protein that is made by hepatocytes in response to inflammation (ie, cytokines). The normal concentration of this protein is 10 mg/L.[1] Postoperative infection can lead to elevation of the CRP level from 40 mg/L to more than 200 mg/L.[1,2] Units for CRP levels vary amongst laboratories, with some reporting as milligrams per deciliter.[1] The ESR is also a measure of inflammation, with a normal ESR considered to be less than 15 to 20 mm/h. In response to inflammation, CRP level is elevated more rapidly than ESR. Similarly, after the source of inflammation is successfully treated, CRP level returns to normal more rapidly than ESR, with a reported elimination half ranging from 2.6 to 9 days.[1,3,4] Kahn and colleagues[5] reported that, in the setting of postoperative spinal wound infection, CRP level is of value in following the response to treatment but that ESR can remain persistently elevated, despite a normal CRP level and clinical evidence of a successfully treated infection. Both the CRP level and ESR are normally elevated after surgery. In one study, after uncomplicated spine surgery, the CRP level and ESRs were noted to peak at 166 mg/L and 68 mm/h on postoperative days 2.7 and 4.2, respectively.[4] Unless a wound infection develops, the CRP level should normalize within 1 to 2 weeks and the ESR should normalize within about 6 weeks.

The incidence of recurrent laryngeal nerve injury is reported to be as high as 3.5% in primary and 9.5% in revision anterior cervical spine surgery.[6] When planning revision anterior cervical spine surgery, it is therefore important to send the patient for vocal cord evaluation by an otolaryngologist to determine if there was an injury to the recurrent laryngeal nerve during the initial procedure. Through either a mirror examination and/or direct laryngoscopy performed in the office setting, the otolaryngologist can determine if there is partial or complete paralysis of the vocal cord ipsilateral to the side of the previous anterior approach. If there is evidence of vocal cord paralysis on the side of the previous anterior cervical surgery, the revision anterior procedure should be performed from the same side to avoid injury to the normal vocal cord. If the vocal cords are normal, then it is preferred that the revision anterior surgery be performed from the contralateral side to avoid scar tissue that can complicate the approach.

When planning revision anterior cervical spine surgery, particularly when anterior instrumentation is present, attention must be given to the esophagus. Although esophageal injury is rare, it is a devastating complication. Esophageal injury can occur either as a result of erosion of existing anterior instrumentation through the esophageal wall or as a result of intraoperative injury. The presence of persistent dysphagia after the initial procedure, prominent anterior instrumentation, and/or anterior instrumentation that is backing out should prompt a preoperative evaluation of the esophagus by an otolaryngologist. A videofluoroscopic swallowing study can assess esophageal function during swallowing and can identify adhesion and possibly perforation at the site of existing instrumentation. Direct esophagoscopy can identify whether or not the instrumentation has eroded through the esophagus. When the preoperative evaluation suggests that the existing anterior instrumentation has compromised the esophageal wall, the otolaryngologist should be consulted for intraoperative assistance during the revision procedure. The risk of intraoperative esophageal injury is elevated in the revision setting. Intraoperative assessment of the integrity of the esophagus can be accomplished using methylene blue. An orogastric tube is placed down the esophagus so that the tip of the tube is within the esophagus at the level of the surgery. The surgeon then applies slight pressure to the esophagus distal to the tube and has the anesthesiologist inject 60 mL of methylene blue/saline. After the solution is injected, the anterior cervical wound is assessed for the presence of the blue solution, the presence of which suggests an esophageal injury.[7]

SPINAL PATHOLOGY REQUIRING REVISION SURGERY

A comprehensive systematic approach is required when a patient presents with recurrent symptoms after prior cervical spine surgery. Surgery performed at the wrong level, gross hardware failure, or instability often requires revision surgery. The presenting signs and symptoms (axial pain, myelopathy, or radiculopathy) guide diagnostic workup and management. Workup of axial neck pain after fusion is best accomplished with CT scan with sagittal and coronal reconstructions to determine the presence or absence of fusion. If symptomatic pseudarthrosis is present, revision surgery may be indicated. If solid fusion is noted, MRI can identify the presence of same and/or adjacent segment degenerative disease, which may be managed conservatively or surgically. CT myelogram and/or MRI can typically identify same or adjacent segment central or foraminal stenosis. Patients with myelopathy typically require revision decompression, whereas those with radiculopathy can be managed nonoperatively or operatively. If MRI is unremarkable, electromyography (EMG) and nerve conduction studies (NCS) are indicated to evaluate for peripheral nerve compression or polyradiculopathies.

Adjacent Segment Disease

Adjacent segment cervical disease (ASD) is noted in roughly 3% of patients per year; however, incidence increases to approximately 25% of patients within the first 10 years after the index fusion procedure is expected.[8] Adjacent segment disease, simply defined, is the development of symptomatic spondylosis and/or disk herniation adjacent to a prior fused level.[8] Presence of clinical symptoms delineates this definition from adjacent segment degeneration, which refers to the presence of degeneration on imaging studies.[9–11] A host of clinical, biomechanical, and basic science reports abound in the literature regarding the cause, nature, and course of the disease. Pivotal to the debate is the question whether degeneration occurs as a result of the natural history in patients at risk for spondylosis or the increased motion and stress at the disc adjacent to a rigid fusion. A combination of factors probably contributes to ASD development, including the increased biomechanical stress placed on the disk space adjacent to a fusion and the natural history of cervical spondylosis in patients known to have such pathology.[12]

Clinical studies primarily concentrate on retrospective reviews with varying imaging modalities to determine adjacent segment degeneration with or without clinical symptoms. Dohler and colleagues[9] found an asymptomatic adjacent level translation of 67% at 27 months of mean follow-up after ACDF. Kyphotic alignment at an operated level might be a risk factor for adjacent segment degeneration. Katsuura and colleagues[10] failed to show differences in Japanese Orthopaedic Association scores before, after, or at final follow-up in patients with or without adjacent segment degeneration. At a long-term 100-month follow-up, Goffin and colleagues[11] showed an incidence of adjacent segment degeneration of 92% correlated poorly with ASD and reoperation (6%). Hilibrand and colleagues[8] noted an annual incidence of ASD of 2.9% with 25% chance at 10-year follow-up. Other studies corroborate these findings and found increased risk of symptomatic ASD when index operation preoperative imaging showed ventral dural compression via

the disk, lending some to recommend inclusion of the adjacent levels at the index operation.[13,14]

In response to increased awareness of ASD, motion-sparing techniques and devices have been advocated, primarily including posterior laminoforaminotomy and cervical disk replacement. Although most studies of ASD pertain to anterior cervical fusion, posterior procedures also experience ASD and degeneration postoperatively. Laminoforaminotomy has been implicated with similar rates of adjacent segment pathology compared with ACDF (50% vs 41% at 4.5-year follow-up) in addition to 3.3% same segment disease at 7-year follow-up.[15,16] This suggests that natural history likely contributes to ASD development after posterior laminoforaminotomy. Clinical studies have varied in results when comparing adjacent segmental motion after arthroplasty with ACDF, with some showing increased motion, no difference, or decreased motion in patients with arthroplasty.[17,18] Clinical outcomes seem to be similar functionally between arthroplasty and single-level ACDF with allograft and plating, although the need for reoperation due to ASD might be lower with arthroplasty.[19]

Presenting symptoms and signs of ASD may include myelopathy- and/or radiculopathy-related complaints. Static and dynamic radiographs may demonstrate changes of spondylosis or degeneration, including disk space narrowing; subchondral end plate sclerosis; osteophyte (anterior, posterior, or uncovertebral) formation; and, less commonly, instability. MRI is the modality of choice to evaluate the discoligamentous structures, when assessing for neural compression correlating with the patient's clinical presentation.

Same Segment Disease (Incomplete ACDF or Disk Arthroplasty)

Same segment disease usually implies inadequate decompression at the levels operated at the index procedure or, in the setting of cervical disk replacement, the recurrence of disease. Revision anterior surgery for inadequate decompression is typically more difficult than the original procedure including dissection through a scar bed with and takedown of prior hardware and bone graft material. To adequately diagnose and treat same segment disease, the physician must be completely versed in the differential diagnoses mimicking compressive cervical lesions. Once an accurate diagnosis is made, use of imaging studies, including static and dynamic radiography, CT, and MRI (occasionally including dynamic studies and oblique views to evaluate for more subtle dynamic compression or foraminal disease), can allow the surgeon to create a comprehensive preoperative plan based on the location of compression, number of levels involved, presence of hard or soft disks, sagittal alignment, presence of retrovertebral pathology or ossification of the posterior longitudinal ligament (PLL), presence of instability, and axial neck pain.[20–22] The surgeon's armamentarium of anterior (ACDF, anterior cervical corpectomy and fusion [ACCF], hybrid ACCF + ACDF), posterior (laminoforaminotomy, laminectomy with fusion, or laminaplasty), or combined procedures can then be appropriately used.

In patients who present with persistence of preoperative symptoms, the treating physician must consider the possible causes, including inaccurate original diagnosis, inadequate decompression, unrecognized preexisting irreversible spinal cord/nerve root, iatrogenic spinal cord/nerve root injury, postoperative instability, adjacent segment disease, and pseudarthrosis. Differential diagnosis for cervical myelopathy includes intracranial, intraspinal, and peripheral nerve disorders such as multiple sclerosis (visual symptoms, facial numbness, migratory neurologic complaints, oligoclonal cerebrospinal fluid [CSF] bands); amyotrophic lateral sclerosis (combined progressive upper and lower motor neuron disease of anterior horn cells); Guillain-Barré syndrome (increased CSF protein in postviral patients with ascending sensorimotor polyneuropathy); pernicious anemia (vitamin B12 deficiency with macrocytic anemia, dorsal column dysfunction); peripheral nerve entrapment disorders of the radial, median, and ulnar nerves (commonly carpal and cubital tunnel syndromes); syringomyelia; irreversible preexisting spinal cord changes; infection; or intraspinal or intracranial tumors. Workup is dictated by thorough history taking, physical examination, and then subsequent imaging (spinal or intracranial CT with/without myelography, MRI) or diagnostic tests (EMG/NCS, CSF analysis, laboratory analysis, and consultation with neurologists as indicated).

CT myelography is excellent for evaluating adequacy of decompression, presence of fusion or pseudarthrosis, graft and hardware location and status, presence of residual bony compression, infolding of redundant ligamentum flavum, and facet arthrosis.[22] MRI can evaluate the status of the spinal cord and quantify myelomalacia and cord atrophy and whether reversible (low-intensity T2 changes) or irreversible (high-intensity focal T2 and low-signal T1 changes or "snake-eye" appearance of anterior horn cells cystic necrosis) changes are present.[23,24] In addition to these MRI signal changes, chronic symptoms for more than 18 months, age more than 60 years, spinal cord transverse area less than 50 mm², and multilevel compression are risk factors for poor outcomes.[25,26] Intraoperative neurologic injury should be noted in the initial records on transcranial motor evoked potentials and somatosensory potentials secondary typically to direct neurologic trauma or hypoperfusion from hypotension.

After defining the offending structures, surgical plan and procedures are chosen based on multiple factors. If compression is located anteriorly, presence of 1- or 2-level disease is best approached with ACDF if any spondylotic or hard disk component is noted with excellent results. If the PLL had not been previously resected, it is recommended in the revision setting to resect the PLL and perform a direct uncovertebral decompression to ensure that the compressive pathology is adequately removed. Patients with multilevel anterior compression with kyphotic alignment must be evaluated for the need to perform a corpectomy versus multilevel ACDF. Multilevel ACDFs provide increased biomechanical stability and increased lordosis but higher risk of pseudarthrosis given more fusion surfaces (ie, up to 47%–56% with 3- and 4-level cases).[27–29] Multilevel ACCF has relatively high fusion rates (ie, 86%–99%) but an increased rate of graft dislodgement that usually necessitates posterior fixation for more than 2-level corpectomies.[30,31] Patients with multilevel (>3 levels) anterior fusions may require posterior supplementary fixation. Compressive lesions located ventrally over multilevels that have neutral or lordotic sagittal alignment can be approached by either laminectomy with fusion (ie, if preexisting instability or axial neck pain is noted) or laminoplasty with or without foraminotomies (ie, when no instability or neck pain exists preoperatively) with good results more than 90% time in appropriately selected patients.[32,33]

The advent of minimally invasive and motion-sparing technologies does not change the primary need for adequate decompression. Compared with ACDF in which posterior osteophytes may be absorbed over time, patients who have undergone cervical disk replacement require a complete osteophyte decompression because motion is preserved.[34,35] Careful attention to detail is also required during foraminotomy. Lehman and Riew[36] recommend dorsally unroofing the nerve by resecting up to 50% of the superior articular facet with or without removal of underlying disks or burring of the uncovertebral joint osteophytes. Given the preservation of motion, osteophytes and compressive pathologic condition can reoccur after cervical disk replacement at the same segment. Diagnosis is complicated by the presence of the prosthesis, which creates artifact on imaging studies. CT myelography can be helpful when trying to diagnose same segment disease after cervical disk replacement. Selective nerve root injections can aid in the diagnosis if questions remain as to which levels are symptomatic. The presence of persistent or recurrent foraminal disease after cervical disk arthroplasty may be amenable to posterior laminoforaminotomy.

Pseudarthrosis

Cervical pseudarthroses are known complications of both anterior and posterior fusions and typically occurring at the caudalmost level. Incidence of pseudarthrosis after single-level ACDF ranges from 0% to 20%, escalating to 40% to 50% for multilevel procedures.[29,37–40] Cervical spine fusion rates vary depending on many factors, including approach (anterior vs posterior), number of levels fused, type of grafting technique (autograft, allograft), presence of deformity, and patient-specific factors (smoking, diabetes, prior history of pseudarthrosis). Planning revision surgery can be complicated by the presence of prior approach-related complications (ie, anterior scarring, recurrent laryngeal nerve injury, and dysphagia). Patients are symptomatic in two-thirds of pseudarthroses, and patients typically complain of axial neck pain, radiculitis, or a combination of recurring or persisting preoperative symptoms.[37] Dynamic

flexion and extension radiographs may show gross instability at the level of pseudarthrosis, screw/rod breakage, migration of instrumentation, and/or haloing of screws. CT scan is the imaging modality of choice when evaluating for presence of pseudarthroses, the status of any instrumentation (ie, loosening, breakage, migration), bone quality, and presence of any offending compressive structures in patients with neurologic symptoms and signs (**Fig. 4**). Intraoperative confirmation of motion at the motion segment, lack of bony bridging trabeculae, and graft resorbtions are suggestive of a pseudarthrosis.

Treatment of pseudarthroses is usually nonoperative in asymptomatic individuals, and up to 30% do not require revision surgery.[41,42] Operative treatment is required for those with unstable/failed hardware and appropriate for those select patients who remain symptomatic despite conservative measures. Treatment of posterior pseudarthrosis can be complicated in the setting of prior decompression because there is an increased risk of incidental durotomy during surgical dissection. In these cases, anterior cervical fusion is preferred. Patients without exposed dura can be approached dorsally, ventrally, or circumferentially depending on the amount of stabilization required to achieve a biomechanically sound construct allowing arthrodesis. Treatment options for anterior pseudarthroses typically involve revision anterior repair,

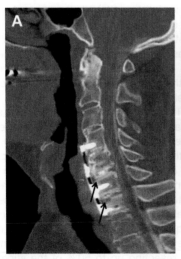 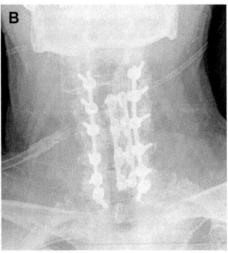

Fig. 4. (*A*) Sagittal midline reconstruction of a cervical CT myelogram in a patient 1 year after anterior cervical discectomy and fusion from C4 to C7 for cervical spondylotic myelopathy. The patient did not improve after the initial operation, has persistent signs and symptoms of myelopathy, and now has persistent axial neck pain. This CT myelogram demonstrates clear pseudarthoses at the C5-6 and C6-7 levels (*black arrows*) as well as persistent stenosis from C4 to T1. (*B*) Postoperative anteroposterior cervical radiograph following a posterior cervical laminectomy and fusion from C3 to T1 in this patient, who after surgery had significant improvement in both his neck pain and myelopathic symptoms.

posterior fusion, or combined anterior/posterior stabilization and fusion. Direct evaluation, removal, and grafting of the pseudarthrosis are possible via revision anterior repair, but difficult dissection through scar tissue beds increases risk of viscus, vessel, or nerve injury as well as increased rates of dysphagia and dysphonia. Anterior repair typically has lower blood loss and shorter hospital stays but lower union rates (45% vs 95%–97%) than posterior procedures.[43,44] Overall, complication rates (mostly wound or graft harvest related) are reported to be slightly higher with posterior surgery.[44]

Surgical technique for successful revision anterior repair or posterior fusion hinges on adequate decompression of neural structures, preparation of a good fusion bed, use of adequate bone graft and/or bone graft substitute, and stable fixation. During revision anterior repair, complete excision of fibrous nonosseous material is required as well as a thorough decompression of the neural elements, especially in patients with signs and/or symptoms of radiculopathy or myelopathy. Iliac crest autograft is a reliable option for grafting in the revision situation. Posterior fusion alone or as part of circumferential stabilization is the authors' treatment of choice as long as anterior hardware and grafts are stable and kyphotic deformity does not exist. This approach provides a high rate of fusion and clinical success, more so than the anterior approach.[42–44] Decompression in most cases consists of laminoforaminotomy at the indicated levels. Kuhns and colleagues[45] demonstrated no difference in patients treated with autogenous iliac crest or local bone graft. Stabilization is typically achieved with posterior lateral mass screw/rod constructs. At the C7 and T1 levels, the authors typically use pedicle screw fixation (see **Fig. 2C**).

Progressive Deformity (Postlaminectomy Kyphosis)

Iatrogenic cervical deformity most often occurs after posterior decompressive procedures involving disruption of the tension band (posterior ligamentous complex), muscular denervation and weakness, and excessive capsulectomy and/or facetectomy.[46–48] Although the deformities can involve both the coronal and sagittal planes, the dominant alignment is typically kyphosis because the center of gravity shifts anteriorly given the weight of the head, muscular weakness, and ligamentous and articular disruptions. Multilevel cervical laminectomies carry a 20% risk, which can be higher in skeletally immature and young adult patients (given incomplete osseous formation, wedging, and relative ligamentous laxity).[49–51] Iatrogenic kyphosis is also increased after laminoplasty secondary to the disruption of the muscular, fascial, and ligamentous structures.[52] Risk factors include increased age, preoperative sagittal kyphotic alignment, poor intraoperative positioning, inadequate grafting techniques or subsidence, and aggressive facetectomies.[53] Clinically, patients typically present with muscular fatigue, neck pain, difficulty maintaining a horizontal gaze, a kyphotic sagittal appearance on lateral observation with the head protruding forward, and possible neurologic symptoms and signs, including myelopathy or radiculopathy.[53] Diagnostic workup radiographs help evaluate coronal imbalance, maximum deformity, and the amount of correction that can be obtained (fixed vs flexible deformity). CT scan is helpful in determining the presence of bony ankylosis dorsally or ventral fusion in patients with fixed deformities as well as in planning surgical corrective maneuvers (**Fig. 5**). MRI is useful for patients with neurologic complaints or signs to determine where decompression is needed as well as to evaluate for and quantify the amount of myelomalacia, cord atrophy, and syringomyelia, which can complicate as well as increase risk of treatment.[53]

The goals of surgical treatment are decompression and protection of neural elements with maintenance of neurologic function, deformity correction, and long-term stabilization via arthrodesis. Treatment algorithm centers on approach selection with a posterior-only, anterior-only, combined anterior-posterior, or posterior-anterior-posterior approach. Determination of a fixed versus flexible deformity is of primary importance. Patients who correct to neutral on full-extension preoperative radiographs can be candidates for either anterior- or posterior-only procedures. If no ventral compressive pathologic condition is noted in a patient with flexible deformity corrected on extension radiographs, posterior arthrodesis with stable lateral mass/pedicle instrumentation yields good results. When patients are extended intraoperatively from a neutral position, appropriate laminoforaminotomies should be performed to prevent iatrogenic root compression. Less often, patients with focal fixed kyphosis without dorsal element ankylosis are candidates for anterior release and reconstruction (via diskectomy [ACDF], corpectomy [ACCF] if retrovertebral compression exists, or a combination of anterior procedures), with correction of 20° possible.[54] If global flexible kyphosis exists, multilevel ACDF is preferred because it allows increased lordotic correction and number of fixation points and, typically, has lower graft dislodgement than a long

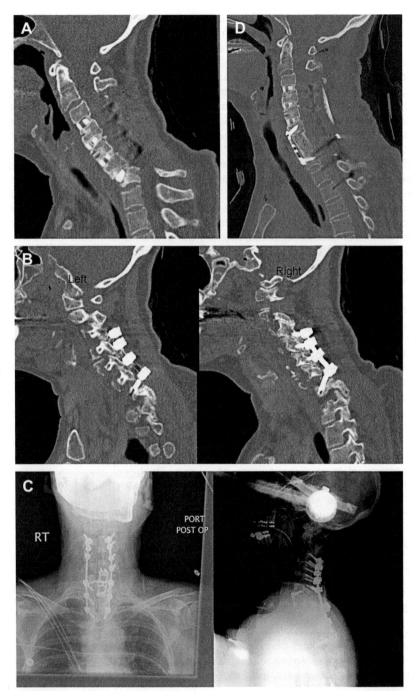

Fig. 5. (*A*) Sagittal midline and (*B*) and left and right parasagittal CT scan reconstructions in a patient 4 months after combined anterior/posterior decompression and fusion from C3 to C7. These CT images demonstrate pullout of the C7 pedicle screws bilaterally with fracture of the pedicles and the development of a significant kyphotic deformity. The graft at C6-C7 has displaced anteriorly and there is a fracture of the C7 vertebral body. The patient underwent a revision anterior C7 corpectomy with use of structural iliac crest allograft bone and anterior instrumentation followed by posterior instrumentation and fusion extended down to the T3 level. This is demonstrated in the postoperative (*C*) anteroposterior (*left*) and lateral (*right*) cervical radiographs and (*D*) a sagittal midline CT scan reconstruction.

corpectomy.[53,55,56] Plating is helpful to prevent graft dislodgement and increase union rates. Combined anterior/posterior approaches are recommended for multilevel revision reconstructions involving 3 or more levels. Riew and colleagues[57] found a high incidence of graft-related complications (ie, 82%) in patients with postlaminectomy kyphosis treated with multilevel ACCF with struts and advocate circumferential stabilization. In the presence of rigid deformity, some investigators advocate preoperative traction in preparation for correction.[56] Fixed anterior deformities either require anterior release followed by posterior stabilization or a posterior transpedicular osteotomy.

Infection

Postoperative infection following cervical spine surgery is relatively rare and occurs more commonly after posterior cervical procedures than anterior cervical procedures. The pathophysiology of postoperative infection involves a combination of bacterial load, spinal implants, and postoperative hematoma that creates an ideal bacterial growth environment. Elucidation of appropriate guidelines and subsequent standards for evaluation, diagnosis, and treatment of postoperative spinal wound infections remains paramount. Vital preoperative, intraoperative, and postoperative risk factors must be recognized to minimize the risk of developing a postoperative infection (**Box 1**). Preoperative and perioperative risk factors in adults include diabetes, alcohol abuse, smoking, history of prior infections, age more than 60 years, and increased surgical time.[58]

Diagnostic workup is described previously remembering that CRP level determination is the most sensitive laboratory test for acute postoperative infection. The combination of pain, hardware loosening, and a rim-enhancing lesion on MRI indicates a delayed postoperative infection. MRI is the imaging study of choice to identify a postoperative abscess (**Fig. 6**). The presence of a deep or superficial fluid collection on MRI along with a clinical picture of an infection (ie, elevated CRP level, ESR, and/or white blood cell count; fever; wound drainage and/or erythema; increased pain; neurologic symptoms) warrants operative irrigation and drainage. Instrumentation can typically be salvaged if no loosening is noted at the time of irrigation and drainage. Every effort is made to retain instrumentation in the setting of postoperative infection until the fusion is solid to avoid the potential for spinal instability. Multiple irrigation and debridements and/or the temporary

---

Box 1
Risk factors for postoperative spinal surgical site infections

Preoperative
- Prior spinal surgery
- ASA>2[a]
- Obesity[a]
- Prophylactic antibiotics (inappropriate timing, clindamycin)[a]
- Diabetes mellitus[a]
- History of prior infections[a]
- Smoking
- Severe acne
- Comorbid PMH (hypothyroid, cardiomyopathy, steroid use, immunosuppression, sickle cell disease, ITP)

Intraoperative
- Surgery longer than 5 hours[a]
- Staged procedures[a]
- More than 10 vertebrae fused
- Blood loss>80 mL/kg
- Two or more residents
- Instrumentation
- Allograft
- Fusion to the sacrum

Postoperative
- Blood transfusion[a]
- Lack of postoperative drains[a]
- High output or distally placed drains (near rectum)

Abbreviations: ASA, American Society of Anesthesiologists classification; ITP, idiopathic thrombotic purpura; PMH, past medical history.
[a] Multivariate risk factor.

---

use of a vacuum-assisted closure dressing may be needed to obtain a healthy-appearing wound that can definitively closed. Definitive closure should be performed over deep and/or superficial drains, depending on the primary location of the infection. Intraoperative cultures should be taken and an infectious disease specialist should be consulted to guide antibiotic therapy. A typical antibiotic regimen for a deep cervical postoperative infection included 6 to 8 weeks of intravenous antibiotics followed by a variable course of postoperative antibiotics. Infectious laboratory work

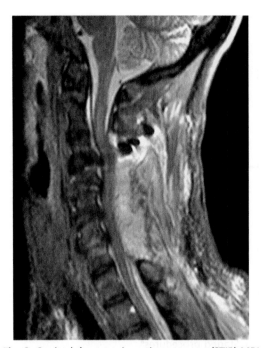

Fig. 6. Sagittal short tau inversion recovery (STIR) MRI image of the cervical spine in a patient who presented to the emergency room 3 weeks after posterior cervical laminectomy and fusion with complaints of fever, chills, and increased neck pain. The MRI demonstrates a large fluid collection in the site of the laminectomy causing significant compression of the spinal cord. This patient was taken for irrigation and debridement of the posterior cervical deep abscess, closed over deep drains, and treated with 6 weeks of intravenous antibiotics. The infection was successfully treated and instrumentation was salvaged.

(ESR and CRP level) should be followed up to ensure successful treatment and resolution of the infection.

SUMMARY

Revision spine surgical procedures typically involve pseudarthrosis, infection, adjacent segment disease, same segment disease, instrumentation failure, and progressive deformity. Systematic evaluation through history taking, physical examination, indicated imaging studies, and laboratory tests can yield accurate diagnoses and detailed preoperative plans for addressing the cause of initial surgical failure. Revision principles are based on adequate decompression of neural elements and mechanical stability via appropriate selection of surgical approach and constructs producing long-term stability with arthrodesis. Although most cases are more complex with the potential for increased complications relative to primary surgery, adherence to fundamental principles allow acceptable clinical outcomes.

REFERENCES

1. Clyne B, Olshaker JS. The C-reactive protein. J Emerg Med 1999;17:1019–25.
2. Jupe D. The acute phase response and laboratory testing. Aust Fam Physician 1996;25:324–9.
3. Young B, Gleeson M, Cripps AW. C-reactive protein: a critical review. Pathology 1991;23:118–24.
4. Mok JM, Pekmezci M, Piper SL, et al. Use of C-reactive protein after spinal surgery: comparison with erythrocyte sedimentation rate as predictor of early postoperative infectious complications. Spine (Phila Pa 1976) 2008;33:415–21.
5. Khan MH, Smith PN, Rao N, et al. Serum C-reactive protein levels correlate with clinical response in patients treated with antibiotics for wound infections after spinal surgery. Spine J 2006;6:311–5.
6. Beutler WJ, Sweeney CA, Connolly PJ. Recurrent laryngeal nerve injury with anterior cervical spine surgery risk with laterality of surgical approach. Spine (Phila Pa 1976) 2001;26:1337–42.
7. Taylor B, Patel AA, Okubadejo GO, et al. Detection of esophageal perforation using intraesophageal dye injection. J Spinal Disord Tech 2006;19: 191–3.
8. Hilibrand AS, Carlson GD, Palumbo MA, et al. Radiculopathy and myelopathy at segments adjacent to the site of a previous anterior cervical arthrodesis. J Bone Joint Surg Am 1999;81:519–28.
9. Dohler JR, Kahn MR, Hughes SP. Instability of the cervical spine after anterior interbody fusion. A study on its incidence and clinical significance in 21 patients. Arch Orthop Trauma Surg 1985;104: 247–50.
10. Katsuura A, Hukuda S, Saruhashi Y, et al. Kyphotic malalignment after anterior cervical fusion is one of the factors promoting the degenerative process in adjacent intervertebral levels. Eur Spine J 2001;10: 320–4.
11. Goffin J, Geusens E, Vantomme N, et al. Long-term follow-up after interbody fusion of the cervical spine. J Spinal Disord Tech 2004;17:79–85.
12. Eck JC, Humphreys SC, Lim TH, et al. Biomechanical study on the effect of cervical spine fusion on adjacent-level intradiscal pressure and segmental motion. Spine (Phila Pa 1976) 2002;27:2431–4.
13. Yue WM, Brodner W, Highland TR. Long-term results after anterior cervical discectomy and fusion with allograft and plating: a 5- to 11-year radiologic and clinical follow-up study. Spine (Phila Pa 1976) 2005;30:2138–44.
14. Ishihara H, Kanamori M, Kawaguchi Y, et al. Adjacent segment disease after anterior cervical interbody fusion. Spine J 2004;4:624–8.

15. Herkowitz HN, Kurz LT, Overholt DP. Surgical management of cervical soft disc herniation. A comparison between the anterior and posterior approach. Spine (Phila Pa 1976) 1990;15:1026–30.

16. Clarke MJ, Ecker RD, Krauss WE, et al. Same-segment and adjacent-segment disease following posterior cervical foraminotomy. J Neurosurg Spine 2007;6:5–9.

17. Pickett GE, Rouleau JP, Duggal N. Kinematic analysis of the cervical spine following implantation of an artificial cervical disc. Spine (Phila Pa 1976) 2005;30:1949–54.

18. Nabhan A, Pape D, Pitzen T, et al. Radiographic analysis of fusion progression following one-level cervical fusion with or without plate fixation. Zentralbl Neurochir 2007;68:133–8.

19. Mummaneni PV, Burkus JK, Haid RW, et al. Clinical and radiographic analysis of cervical disc arthroplasty compared with allograft fusion: a randomized controlled clinical trial. J Neurosurg Spine 2007;6:198–209.

20. Humphreys SC, An HS, Eck JC, et al. Oblique MRI as a useful adjunct in evaluation of cervical foraminal impingement. J Spinal Disord 1998;11:295–9.

21. Cannada LK, Scherping SC, Yoo JU, et al. Pseudoarthrosis of the cervical spine: a comparison of radiographic diagnostic measures. Spine (Phila Pa 1976) 2003;28:46–51.

22. Ploumis A, Mehbod A, Garvey T, et al. Prospective assessment of cervical fusion status: plain radiographs versus CT-scan. Acta Orthop Belg 2006;72:342–6.

23. Chen CJ, Lyu RK, Lee ST, et al. Intramedullary high signal intensity on T2-weighted MR images in cervical spondylotic myelopathy: prediction of prognosis with type of intensity. Radiology 2001;221:789–94.

24. Mizuno J, Nakagawa H, Inoue T, et al. Clinicopathological study of "snake-eye appearance" in compressive myelopathy of the cervical spinal cord. J Neurosurg 2003;99:162–8.

25. Naderi S, Ozgen S, Pamir MN, et al. Cervical spondylotic myelopathy: surgical results and factors affecting prognosis. Neurosurgery 1998;43:43–9 [discussion: 9–50].

26. Wada E, Yonenobu K, Suzuki S, et al. Can intramedullary signal change on magnetic resonance imaging predict surgical outcome in cervical spondylotic myelopathy? Spine (Phila Pa 1976) 1999;24:455–61 [discussion: 62].

27. Emery SE, Bohlman HH, Bolesta MJ, et al. Anterior cervical decompression and arthrodesis for the treatment of cervical spondylotic myelopathy. Two to seventeen-year follow-up. J Bone Joint Surg Am 1998;80:941–51.

28. Bolesta MJ, Rechtine GR 2nd, Chrin AM. Three- and four-level anterior cervical discectomy and fusion with plate fixation: a prospective study. Spine (Phila Pa 1976) 2000;25:2040–4 [discussion: 5–6].

29. Papadopoulos EC, Huang RC, Girardi FP, et al. Three-level anterior cervical discectomy and fusion with plate fixation: radiographic and clinical results. Spine (Phila Pa 1976) 2006;31:897–902.

30. Zdeblick TA, Hughes SS, Riew KD, et al. Failed anterior cervical discectomy and arthrodesis. Analysis and treatment of thirty-five patients. J Bone Joint Surg Am 1997;79:523–32.

31. Vaccaro AR, Falatyn SP, Scuderi GJ, et al. Early failure of long segment anterior cervical plate fixation. J Spinal Disord 1998;11:410–5.

32. Herkowitz HN. A comparison of anterior cervical fusion, cervical laminectomy, and cervical laminoplasty for the surgical management of multiple level spondylotic radiculopathy. Spine (Phila Pa 1976) 1988;13:774–80.

33. Herkowitz HN. Cervical laminaplasty: its role in the treatment of cervical radiculopathy. J Spinal Disord 1988;1:179–88.

34. An HS, Evanich CJ, Nowicki BH, et al. Ideal thickness of Smith-Robinson graft for anterior cervical fusion. A cadaveric study with computed tomographic correlation. Spine (Phila Pa 1976) 1993;18:2043–7.

35. Anderson PA, Sasso RC, Riew KD. Update on cervical artificial disk replacement. Instr Course Lect 2007;56:237–45.

36. Lehman RA Jr, Riew KD. Thorough decompression of the posterior cervical foramen. Instr Course Lect 2007;56:301–9.

37. Bohlman HH, Emery SE, Goodfellow DB, et al. Robinson anterior cervical discectomy and arthrodesis for cervical radiculopathy. Long-term follow-up of one hundred and twenty-two patients. J Bone Joint Surg Am 1993;75:1298–307.

38. Newman M. The outcome of pseudarthrosis after cervical anterior fusion. Spine (Phila Pa 1976) 1993;18:2380–2.

39. Wang JC, McDonough PW, Endow KK, et al. Increased fusion rates with cervical plating for two-level anterior cervical discectomy and fusion. Spine (Phila Pa 1976) 2000;25:41–5.

40. Wang JC, McDonough PW, Kanim LE, et al. Increased fusion rates with cervical plating for three-level anterior cervical discectomy and fusion. Spine (Phila Pa 1976) 2001;26:643–6 [discussion: 6–7].

41. Farey ID, McAfee PC, Davis RF, et al. Pseudarthrosis of the cervical spine after anterior arthrodesis. Treatment by posterior nerve-root decompression, stabilization, and arthrodesis. J Bone Joint Surg Am 1990;72:1171–7.

42. Brodsky AE, Khalil MA, Sassard WR, et al. Repair of symptomatic pseudoarthrosis of anterior cervical

fusion. Posterior versus anterior repair. Spine (Phila Pa 1976) 1992;17:1137–43.

43. Lowery GL, Swank ML, McDonough RF. Surgical revision for failed anterior cervical fusions. Articular pillar plating or anterior revision? Spine (Phila Pa 1976) 1995;20:2436–41.

44. Carreon L, Glassman SD, Campbell MJ. Treatment of anterior cervical pseudoarthrosis: posterior fusion versus anterior revision. Spine J 2006;6:154–6.

45. Kuhns CA, Geck MJ, Wang JC, et al. An outcomes analysis of the treatment of cervical pseudarthrosis with posterior fusion. Spine (Phila Pa 1976) 2005; 30:2424–9.

46. Zdeblick TA, Zou D, Warden KE, et al. Cervical stability after foraminotomy. A biomechanical in vitro analysis. J Bone Joint Surg Am 1992;74: 22–7.

47. Nowinski GP, Visarius H, Nolte LP, et al. A biomechanical comparison of cervical laminaplasty and cervical laminectomy with progressive facetectomy. Spine (Phila Pa 1976) 1993;18: 1995–2004.

48. Kumaresan S, Yoganandan N, Pintar FA, et al. Finite element modeling of cervical laminectomy with graded facetectomy. J Spinal Disord 1997;10:40–6.

49. Lonstein JE. Post-laminectomy kyphosis. Clin Orthop Relat Res 1977;(128):93–100.

50. Yasuoka S, Peterson HA, MacCarty CS. Incidence of spinal column deformity after multilevel laminectomy in children and adults. J Neurosurg 1982;57:441–5.

51. Kaptain GJ, Simmons NE, Replogle RE, et al. Incidence and outcome of kyphotic deformity following laminectomy for cervical spondylotic myelopathy. J Neurosurg 2000;93:199–204.

52. Hosalkar HS, Pill SG, Sun PP, et al. Progressive spinal lordosis after laminoplasty in a child with thoracic neuroblastoma. J Spinal Disord Tech 2002;15:79–83.

53. Albert TJ, Vacarro A. Postlaminectomy kyphosis. Spine (Phila Pa 1976) 1998;23:2738–45.

54. Steinmetz MP, Kager CD, Benzel EC. Ventral correction of postsurgical cervical kyphosis. J Neurosurg 2003;98:1–7.

55. Zdeblick TA, Bohlman HH. Cervical kyphosis and myelopathy. Treatment by anterior corpectomy and strut-grafting. J Bone Joint Surg Am 1989;71: 170–82.

56. Herman JM, Sonntag VK. Cervical corpectomy and plate fixation for postlaminectomy kyphosis. J Neurosurg 1994;80:963–70.

57. Riew KD, Hilibrand AS, Palumbo MA, et al. Anterior cervical corpectomy in patients previously managed with a laminectomy: short-term complications. J Bone Joint Surg Am 1999;81:950–7.

58. Fang A, Hu SS, Endres N, et al. Risk factors for infection after spinal surgery. Spine (Phila Pa 1976) 2005;30:1460–5.

Minimally Invasive Approaches to the Cervical Spine

Paul C. Celestre, MD[a],*, Pablo R. Pazmiño, MD[b],
Mark M. Mikhael, MD[a], Christopher F. Wolf, MD[a],
Lacey A. Feldman, BA[c], Carl Lauryssen, MD[c],
Jeffrey C. Wang, MD[a]

KEYWORDS

- Minimally invasive • Cervical spine
- Foraminotomy • Lateral mass screw

The surgical management of cervical radiculopathy has evolved considerably over the past decades; however, no surgical treatment is without associated morbidity or limitations. Traditional techniques of treating patients with radiculopathy from cervical spondylosis have relied on posterior, anterior, and now oblique-based approaches. Minimally invasive approaches and surgical techniques are becoming increasingly popular for the treatment of a variety of cervical spine disorders. Commonly accepted tenants of minimally invasive spine surgery include smaller incisions, paramedian approaches, less dissection and muscle stripping, the use of the operating microscope, specialized retractors and instruments, and an increased reliance on fluoroscopic guidance. The goals of minimally invasive spine surgery are decreased iatrogenic muscle injury, less postoperative pain, and faster recuperation.

The popularity of minimally invasive approaches to the spine has increased proportionally to our understanding of the benefits of these techniques. It is known that traditional open exposures cause iatrogenic muscle injury.[1] Minimally invasive techniques were initially introduced to treat lumbar spine disorders[2] and have been demonstrated to have equivalent outcomes to traditional open procedures.[3]

Fessler and Khoo[4] reported improved postoperative pain with decreased blood loss in a series of patients undergoing minimally invasive cervical foraminal decompression. Two recent prospective, randomized clinical trials comparing minimally invasive posterior cervical foraminotomy with traditional open foraminotomy[5] or anterior cervical discectomy and fusion[6] have demonstrated that minimally invasive techniques can result in smaller incisions, less postoperative pain, and equivalent clinical outcomes.

There is no prospective literature available comparing arthrodesis with lateral mass screws placed in a minimally invasive versus open manner. Wang

Disclosures: PCC, MMM, CFW, LAF: none. PRP is a consultant for Lanx and a clinical instructor for Baxano. CL is a clinical instructor for Ioflex/Baxano and is a consultant for Alphatech, Amedica, Benvenue Medical, Cardo Medical, Crosstree, Dallen Medical, Depuy Spine, Globus, Graphic Surgery, Impliant, INCAS, Intrinsic Therapeutics, K2M, Medtronic-Kyhpon, Orthocon, Osteotech, Paradigm, Pioneer, Replication Medical, Spinal Elements, Spinal Motion, Spinal Kinetics, Spineology, SpineView, Surgitech, and Tissuelink. JCW has a financial relationship or receives royalties from the following companies: Aesculap, Alphatec, Amedica, Biomet, Medtronic Sofamor Danek, Osprey, SeaSpine, Stryker, and Zimmer.

[a] Department of Orthopaedic Surgery, UCLA Comprehensive Spine Center, 1250 16th Street, Suite 745, Santa Monica, CA 90404, USA
[b] SpineCal, 2730 Wilshire Boulevard, Suite 500, Santa Monica, CA 90403, USA
[c] Tower Orthopaedics and Neurosurgical Spine Institute, 8670 Wilshire Boulevard, Suite 200, Beverly Hills, CA 90210, USA
* Corresponding author.
E-mail address: pcelestre@mednet.ucla.edu

Orthop Clin N Am 43 (2012) 137–147
doi:10.1016/j.ocl.2011.08.007
0030-5898/12/$ – see front matter © 2012 Elsevier Inc. All rights reserved.

and Levi[7] reported the successful use of minimally invasive lateral mass screws in 18 patients; however, it is important to note that 2 of these patients required conversion to an open procedure because of an inability to visualize the caudal level.

Anterior cervical neuroforaminal decompression without fusion via a transuncal approach[8,9] is a useful technique in the treatment of cervical radiculopathy while preserving the intervertebral disk and providing complete decompression of the exiting nerve root. Furthermore, anterior approaches offer a direct route to ventral radiculopathy, which can be difficult to address from a posterior approach. Anterior cervical foraminotomy without discectomy potentially leads to decreased operating time, no need for immobilization or hardware, and minimal hospital stay.

Patient interest in minimally invasive cervical spine surgery has expanded dramatically and at a greater rate than medical evidence in support of such techniques. Patient demand for minimally invasive surgery must be tempered by a careful evaluation of patient anatomy and an honest appraisal of a surgeon's experience and ability. Ultimately, a well-performed, thorough open surgery will be more successful than an inadequate minimally invasive operation. In this article, the authors detail minimally invasive approaches to the posterior cervical spine with explanations of both minimally invasive posterior cervical foraminotomy and lateral mass screw placement and describe the technique of minimally invasive anterior cervical foraminotomy.

INDICATIONS

Minimally invasive approaches to the cervical spine have a variety of uses in the treatment of disorders of the cervical spine. Minimally invasive posterior cervical foraminotomy is indicated for the treatment of cervical radiculopathy associated with isolated foraminal stenosis with a soft disk herniation and for the treatment of persistent radicular symptoms following an anterior procedure. Moreover, minimally invasive lateral mass screw fixation can be used to achieve cervical arthrodesis in the setting of subaxial instability and to augment a contemporaneous or prior anterior cervical fusion. Indications for minimally invasive anterior cervical foraminotomy are limited to cervical radiculopathy but include both bilateral radiculopathy and multilevel foraminal stenosis.

CONTRAINDICATIONS

Minimally invasive approaches to the cervical spine are contraindicated in patients with cervical myelopathy secondary to central canal stenosis. Additionally, patients with severely degenerative anatomy, an aberrant course of the vertebral artery (VA), or hypoplasia of the lateral masses are not candidates for minimally invasive lateral mass screw fixation. Minimally invasive approaches to the cervical spine for arthrodesis must be used with extreme caution in trauma patients. Anterior cervical foraminotomy is contraindicated for patients with ossification of the posterior longitudinal ligament, myelopathy, vascular abnormalities, or predominantly significant neck pain. A thorough review of patients' preoperative imaging and knowledge of the course of the VA is mandatory for all anterior procedures. Surgeon inexperience with minimally invasive techniques is an absolute contraindication to minimally invasive cervical spine surgery.

SURGICAL TECHNIQUE
Approach and Technique for Unilateral Posterior Foraminotomy

A minimally invasive approach to the cervical spine can use either a paramedian or midline incision depending on the surgical plan. Paramedian skin incisions are ideal for unilateral foraminotomy but less suited for bilateral procedures or when lateral mass screws will be placed. In such instances, the authors recommend a midline skin incision with two separate paramedian fascial incisions.

To perform a unilateral, single level foraminotomy, patients are positioned prone with the head held in a Mayfield 3-point skull fixation clamp (Integra, Plainsboro, New Jersey). The authors do not typically use monitoring, such as transcranial motor-evoked potentials or somatosensory-evoked potentials, for foraminotomies. The skin is typically injected before incision with a solution of local anesthetic with epinephrine to decrease the inhalational anesthesia requirement and improve hemostasis. Intraoperative fluoroscopy is essential to ensure proper level selection. A 15-mm longitudinal paramedian skin incision is made 5 mm off midline toward the affected side directly centered over the operative level. Dissection is carried straight down to the fascia with electrocautery. A longitudinal fascial incision of equivalent length is then made, and the surgeon's finger is used both to bluntly dissect directly down through the paraspinal muscles to the lateral masses and facet joint of the affected level and to preliminarily clear soft tissue from these structures.

Depending on the retractor system, an initial dilator is then inserted onto the lateral mass and fluoroscopy is used to again confirm the correct level. The dilator can be used as a wanded to help clear soft tissue from the lateral masses and facet joints and to create a potential space in the paraspinal muscles for the tubular retractor. Serial dilators are then inserted, and fluoroscopy is again used to confirm that they remain seated on bone over the operative level. The final dilator is then followed by the tubular retractor itself, which is placed over the final dilator and locked into place. The importance of confirming and reconfirming the correct level cannot be overemphasized because migration of the retractors is common, potentially leading to a wrong-level surgery.

The retractor is then connected to a flexible mounting system and expanded to provide access to the lateral masses and facet joint. At this point, the operative microscope or endoscope is brought in to facilitate visualization and illumination. Electrocautery is used to clear any remaining muscle off of the lateral masses and facet joint. The medial and lateral margins of the lateral masses are key landmarks that must be completely visualized. Dissection should not be carried beyond the lateral margin of the lateral masses because significant bleeding can be encountered, obscuring visualization and increasing the difficulty of the operation.

After the lateral masses and facet joint have been adequately exposed, a final intraoperative radiograph is taken to confirm the correct level before beginning the foraminotomy. The medial half of the inferior articular process of the cephalad vertebra is resected with a 2-mm matchstick high-speed burr. A small amount of lamina of both the superior and inferior vertebra is also routinely removed with the burr to facilitate the identification of the ligamentum flavum. A rent is made in the ligamentum flavum by inserting a short blunt nerve hook into the facet joint, thus, gaining access to the epidural space and then pulling up gently on the ligamentum flavum. A 1-mm Kerrison punch is then used to resect the lateral ligamentum flavum to expose the shining cartilage of the superior articular process of the caudad vertebra. The medial one-third to one-half of the superior articular process is then subtotally resected with the burr, leaving only a thin shell of ventral cortical bone. A short, blunt nerve hook is then inserted into the foramen to create space between the nerve root and this shell of bone. A Kerrison punch or fine curette can be used to remove the remaining cortex of the superior articular facet taking care to prevent injury to the exiting nerve root. Surgifoam (Ethicon, Somerville, New Jersey) or similar hemostatic agents are used liberally during the procedure to maintain a dry operating field and to optimum visualization.

If ventral soft disk material is to be removed, the exiting nerve root can be mobilized superiorly with a short, blunt nerve hook to expose the disk herniation. Great care must be taken to prevent injury to the anterior motor branch, which can be mistaken for disk material.

The described technique can also be used to perform unilateral foraminotomies at multiple levels. Up to 3 sequential foramina may be decompressed via a single paramedian skin incision of 30 mm in this fashion. Exposure is performed in a similar fashion to the technique described for a single-level foraminotomy with a few modifications.

For multilevel foraminotomies, the incision and tubular dilators should be centered on the lateral mass one level above the lowest operative level. The initial dilator should be more aggressively wanded in a cephalad-caudad direction to create a path for the tubular retractor through the paraspinal muscles. Although many retractors are available, a skirted retractor may be advantageous to facilitate visualization in the setting of multilevel surgery (**Figs. 1** and **2**).

Single and multilevel foraminotomies are typically performed on an outpatient basis. Infiltration of the skin with a long-acting anesthetic before termination of the operation helps to decrease immediate postoperative pain. The authors do not routinely discharge patients with a cervical collar. Muscle spasms are common after muscle-splitting approaches and the authors routinely send patients home with an antispasmodic, such as methocarbamol.

Approach and Technique for Bilateral Foraminotomy and Lateral Mass Screw Placement

For minimally invasive bilateral cervical foraminotomies or arthrodesis via lateral mass screw fixation, the authors routinely use a midline posterior cervical incision. The incision, particularly when lateral mass screw fixation is part of the surgical plan, needs 30 to 40 mm in length to facilitate retractor placement. Before incision, the skin is infiltrated with a local anesthetic with epinephrine to assist in hemostasis. Intraoperative fluoroscopy is used to check and recheck the position of the retractor at multiple points in the case to ensure the correct level of operation.

For single-level procedures, fluoroscopy is used to center the incision over the operative level. Dissection is carried down to the fascia with electrocautery and the fascia is cleared 8 mm in each direction off midline. The skin incision is then mobilized to one side and a longitudinal fascial incision is made 5 mm off midline. The surgeon's finger is used to bluntly dissect through the paraspinal muscles down to the lateral masses. The initial dilator is used to preliminarily clear soft

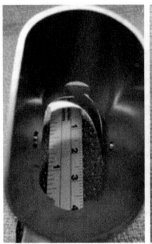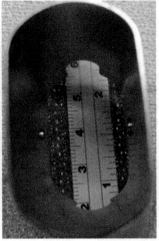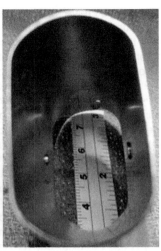

Fig. 1. View through skirted minimally invasive retractor demonstrating 7.5-cm excursion.

tissues from the boney structures and to create a potential space for the retractor.

As discussed previously, a skirted retractor is ideal for multilevel surgeries and especially when lateral mass screw fixation is to be used (see **Figs. 1** and **2**). Once the retractor has been docked over the final dilator and secured to the table, the operating microscope is brought in and electrocautery is used to expose the lateral aspect of the lamina and the medial and lateral extent of the lateral masses to provide anatomic landmarks for lateral mass screws. Care must be taken to limit dissection beyond the lateral extent of the lateral masses to limit bleeding. Minimally invasive foraminotomy then proceeds as described previously.

To place subaxial lateral mass screws via a tubular retractor, the retractor should be oriented approximately 15° to 20° cephalad to facilitate proper trajectory of the screws. It is possible to perform a foraminotomy through a retractor with this orientation, thus, decreasing repositioning of the retractor. After the lateral mass to be instrumented has been completely visualized, the starting point for the screw is found at the midpoint of the lateral mass in the cephalad-caudad direction and 1 mm medial to the midpoint of the lateral mass in the medial-lateral plane. A 2-mm matchstick burr is used to make a pilot hole for the drill.

A drill appropriate for the implant system is brought into the field. The authors routinely use a drill and soft tissue guide with a preset 14-mm stop to prevent anterior cortical penetration. The trajectory for the screw is 15° cephalad for the axial plane and 30° lateral from the sagittal plane.

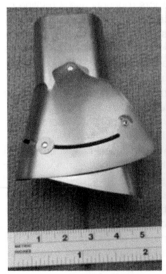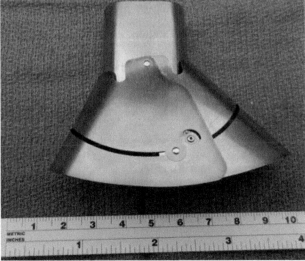

Fig. 2. Skirted minimally invasive retractor in closed versus deployed position.

A ball-tipped probe is used to palpate for cortical breaches and the drill hole is then tapped and again palpated with the ball-tipped probe. Surgifoam (Ethicon, Somerville, New Jersey) is used to control bleeding from the hole, and the screw is then placed and confirmed with fluoroscopy. The authors recommend proceeding from the most cephalad level inferiorly so that the screw heads do not interfere with the trajectory of adjacent screws. Finally, a suitable rod is brought into the field, locked into place with setscrews, and the lateral masses of the vertebrae to be fused are decorticated with a high-speed burr. The wound is irrigated, the bone graft is packed around the lateral masses, the retractor is withdrawn, and the fascia is closed with an absorbable suture. The skin incision is then retracted to the contralateral side and an identical operation is then performed on the if bilateral fixation is desired.

Patients undergoing minimally invasive lateral mass screw arthrodesis are typically placed in an Aspen collar (Aspen Medical Products, Irvine, CA, USA) for 2 to 4 weeks postoperatively. The use of local anesthetic at the conclusion of the operation helps to decrease postoperative pain. These patients are typically observed overnight and leave the following morning. They are placed on antispasmodics immediately postoperatively to decrease muscle spasms.

Anterior Cervical Foraminotomy

Surgical planning concentrates on a thorough evaluation of the lateral one-third of the vertebral unit. To thoroughly assess this area, preoperative diagnostic imaging should include anteroposterior, lateral, flexion-extension, and oblique radiographs of the cervical spine and magnetic resonance imaging (MRI) beforehand. Computed tomography scans are extremely useful to evaluate the extent of bony pathology. Special attention should be made to the relationship between the pathology and 4 key anatomic landmarks: longus colli (LC), uncinate process (UP), VA, and neural elements (N) (**Fig. 3**).

Positioning is similar to that of a standard anterior discectomy with patients in the supine position on a radiolucent table. Because the cervical disk naturally inclines cephalad in the anteroposterior direction, further extension of the cervical spine with bolsters is avoided during patient positioning. Longitudinal traction is not necessary but it may be necessary to tape the patients' shoulders down to visualize the more caudal levels. Preoperative lateral fluoroscopy is used to determine the skin incision, which is made in a skin fold when possible. The surgical technique uses a standard ipsilateral Smith Robinson approach to the vertebral level and side responsible for the radicular pain. The lateral one-third of the vertebral column is delineated with the mobilization of the LC and the placement of retractors in standard fashion. Next the medial and lateral bony margins of the UP are delineated with a combination of electrocautery, kittner dissection, and a freer elevator. The appropriate level is reconfirmed with fluoroscopy and either a minimally invasive tubular retractor or self-retaining retractors are placed deep to the lateral LC and esophagus. Exposure is complete when the UP with the lateral thirds of the cranial and caudal vertebral bodies and disk are within the visual field (**Fig. 3**). In this scenario, multiple adjacent levels can easily be managed from the same skin incision. Because of the potential

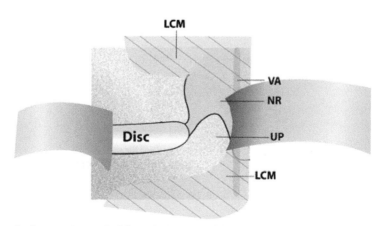

Fig. 3. Key landmarks for anterior cervical foraminotomy. LCM, Longus Coli Muscle; VA, Vertebal Artery; UP, Uncinate Process; NR, Nerve Root.

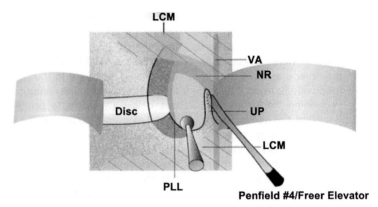

Fig. 4. Protection of the Vertebral Artery.

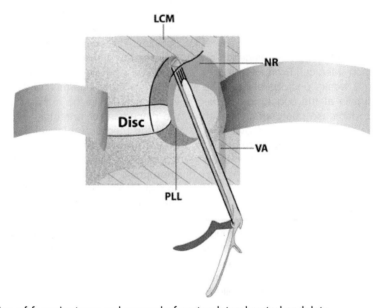

Fig. 5. Progression of foraminotomy and removal of posterolateral rostral endplate.

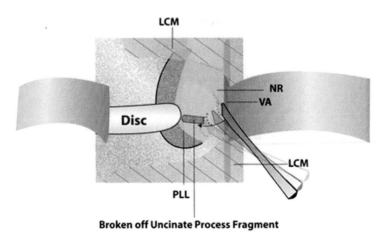

Fig. 6. Removal of UP fragment with Freer elevator.

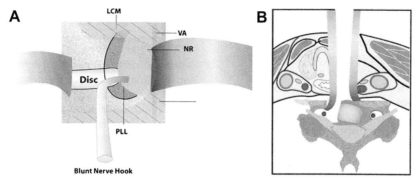

Fig. 7. (*A*) Nerve hook used to check completion of anterior foraminotomy. (*B*) Axial view of complete anterior foraminotomy.

damage to neural and vascular structures, the remainder of the procedure is performed under microscopic magnification. Loupe magnification is suboptimal for visualization and illumination.

A Penfield #4 is used to dissect the lateral margin of the UP of the caudal vertebral body from its investing LC and soft tissue attachments. Hugging the lateral border of the uncinate, dissect a soft tissue plane to place a Penfield #4 between the uncinate and the VA. Once complete, the concave curve of the Penfield #4 should be along the uncinate's lateral margin. This placement serves as an internal metallic medial barrier to the VA (see **Fig. 4**). Next resection of the UP is performed using a long-handled high-speed drill with an AM8 ball-shaped diamond-cutting burr (Anspach, Palm Beach Gardens, Florida/Midas Rex Legend, Fort Worth, Texas). A 6-mm circle of bone is drilled away, while maintaining a 1- to 2-mm margin of bone between the drill and the Penfield #4 (see **Fig. 4**). The drilling is negotiated along the anterolateral course of the UP with judicious saline rinsing and the intermittent placement of bone wax along any bleeding cancellous margins. Fluoroscopic guidance may initially be used to ascertain trajectory and depth. If desired, a wider margin can be obtained by resecting a thin lateral margin of the disk itself to acquire a paracentral disk fragment. The approach vector should be inclined cephalad based on preoperative planning to reach the N posteriorly. A straightforward vector trajectory should be avoided because this would stray toward the superior pedicle margin and away from the foramen. Drilling is advanced judiciously along the posterior cortical uncinate bed and posterolateral rostral endplate. Next the posterior longitudinal ligament (PLL) is identified and a plane is developed between the back of the vertebral body and the PLL. Using a combination of microsect curettage with a 1.0-, 1.5-, or 2.0-mm Kerrison rongeur all overlying bony

margins, osteophytic spurs, cartilage, periosteum, and the lateral margin of the posterior longitudinal ligament are resected from the underlying nerve root (**Fig. 5**). The lateral uncinate wall is thinned with a diamond-tipped burr until a fragment of cortical bone remains, which can be removed near its base by snapping it off from lateral to medial with a Penfield #4 or a Freer elevator (**Fig. 6**). Some investigators prefer to leave this margin as a landmark and protective layer for the underlying VA.[10] As with all minimally invasive procedures, meticulous hemostasis is essential, and control of epidural bleeding or drainage from the anterior internal venous plexus is obtained with a combination of bipolar cautery, gelfoam, and Floseal hemostatic matrix (Baxter Health care Corporation, Deerfield, Illinois).

At this point, the path of the nerve root is decompressed along its length from its emergence near

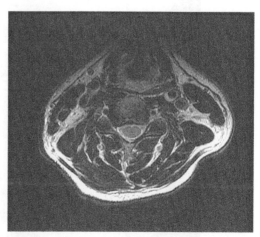

Fig. 8. Preoperative axial MRI of 54-year-old man with right C5 radiculopathy treated with minimally invasive foraminotomy.

the cord to its lateral extent behind the VA. A short, blunt nerve hook is passed along the nerve through the now patent foramina to ensure that all disk fragments have been withdrawn and that an adequate decompression has been performed (**Fig. 7**A and B). Great care must be taken not to retract the root or place further pressure on the already compromised root during the procedure because this may predispose to neurologic injury.

CASE PRESENTATIONS
Case 1

A 54-year-old, right-hand dominant man presented with complaints of 6 months of right lateral arm pain and weakness with overhead activities. He had exhausted all conservative measures, including nonsteroidal antiinflammatory drugs (NSAIDs), physical therapy, and oral steroids over an 8-week period. An MRI demonstrated right C 4/5 foraminal

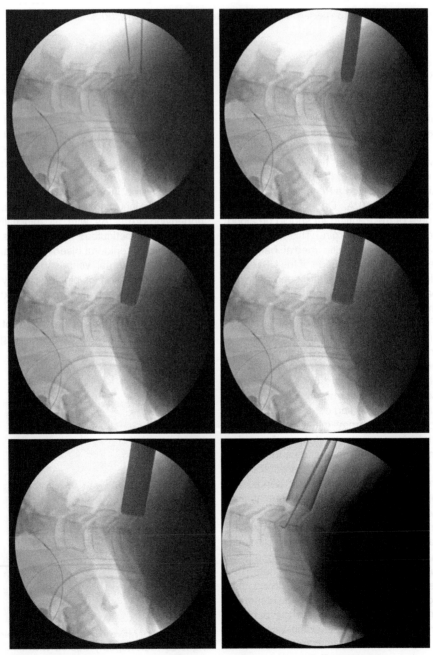

Fig. 9. Sequence of dilation and minimally invasive foraminotomy using tubular retractor.

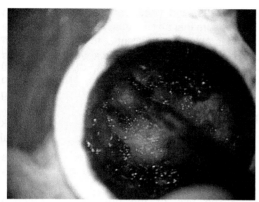

Fig. 10. Intraoperative photograph demonstrating operating microscope view through a tubular retractor and a nerve hook in foramen.

stenosis (**Fig. 8**). The patient was treated with a minimally invasive foraminotomy with a tubular dilator (**Figs. 9** and **10**). The patient remained symptom free at his 3-month follow-up. Postoperative

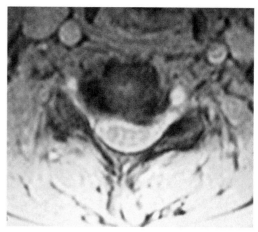

Fig. 12. Preoperative axial MRI demonstrating severe foraminal stenosis at cervical 5/6.

flexion-extension radiographs were obtained and did not show any evidence of instability.

Case 2

A 53-year-old, right-hand dominant man presented with a 9-month history of intractable radiculopathy and weakness in a C6 distribution. He described 90% radicular arm pain and minimal

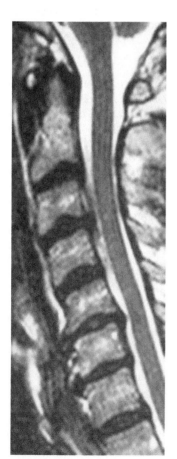

Fig. 11. Preoperative sagittal MRI in a patient with severe foraminal stenosis at cervical 5/6 and predominant right-sided radiculopathy.

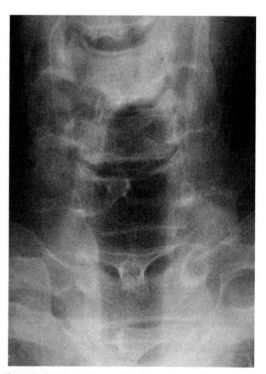

Fig. 13. Postoperative anteroposterior radiograph demonstrating completed right-sided anterior foraminotomy at cervical 5/6.

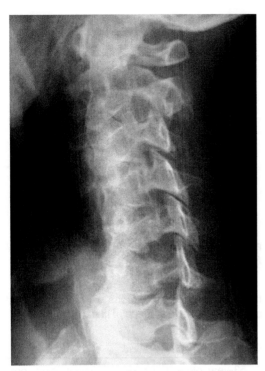

Fig. 14. Postoperative oblique radiograph demonstrating completed right-sided anterior foraminotomy at cervical 5/6.

10% axial neck pain. Despite a prolonged course of conservative management, which included NSAIDs, traction, chiropractic management, physical therapy, oral steroids, epidurals, and selective nerve root blocks, he presented with intractable arm pain and commensurate weakness in a C6 distribution. A preoperative MRI demonstrated right more than left-sided C5/6 foraminal stenosis (**Figs. 11** and **12**). The patient underwent a right-sided C5/6 anterior foraminotomy. The patient remains symptom free at his 2-year follow-up appointment with flexion-extension radiographs, which demonstrate no evidence of any instability. Postoperative anteroposterior and oblique radiographs (**Figs. 13** and **14**) demonstrate the foraminotomy aperture.

SUMMARY

Enthusiasm over minimally invasive spine surgery has been based on the theoretical benefits of smaller incisions and decreased soft tissue stripping, blood loss, postoperative pain, and possibly hospital stays. Minimally invasive approaches to the cervical spine can be used to treat a wide range of pathologic conditions, including radiculopathy secondary to foraminal stenosis, cervical spondylosis, and pseudoarthrosis. The surgeon must ensure that any minimally invasive procedure provides at least equivalent outcomes to an open procedure. Patient selection is key to the success of any operation, and patient safety and satisfaction are the priorities.

TIPS AND PEARLS

- Patient selection is critical for success with minimally invasive techniques, patient desire for a minimally invasive operation is not in itself an indication.
- The use of the operating microscope greatly facilitates illumination and visualization when using tubular retractors.
- The judicious use of intraoperative fluoroscopy is critical to prevent wrong-level surgery.
- Adequate exposure and meticulous hemostasis are essential components to a successful operation.
- A well-performed, thorough open surgery will always be more successful than an inadequate minimally invasive operation.

REFERENCES

1. Styf JR, Willén J. The effects of external compression by three different retractors on pressure in the erector spine muscles during and after posterior lumbar spine surgery in humans. Spine 1998;23: 354–8.
2. Hermantin FU, Peters T, Quartararo L, et al. A prospective, randomized study comparing the results of open discectomy with those of video-assisted arthroscopic microdiscectomy. J Bone Joint Surg Am 1999;81:958–65.
3. Franke J, Greiner-Perth R, Boehm H, et al. Comparison of a minimally invasive procedure versus standard microscopic discotomy: a prospective randomized controlled clinical trial. Eur Spine J 2009;18:992–1000.
4. Fessler RG, Khoo LT. Minimally invasive cervical microendoscopic foraminotomy: an initial clinical experience. Neurosurgery 2002;51:S37–45.
5. Kim KT, Kim YB. Comparison between open procedure and tubular retractor assisted procedure for cervical radiculopathy: results of a randomized controlled study. J Korean Med Sci 2009;24:649–53.
6. Ruetten S, Komp M, Merk H, et al. Full-endoscopic cervical posterior foraminotomy for the operation of lateral disc herniations using 5.9-mm endoscopes: a prospective, randomized, controlled study. Spine 2008;33:940–8.
7. Wang MY, Levi A. Minimally invasive lateral mass screw fixation in the cervical spine: initial clinical

experience with long-term follow up. Neurosurgery 2006;58:907–12.

8. Jho HD. Microsurgical anterior cervical foraminotomy: a new approach to cervical disc herniation. J Neurosurg 1996;84:155–60.

9. Jho HD. Spinal cord decompression via microsurgical anterior foraminotomy for spondylotic cervical myelopathy. Minim Invasive Neurosurg 1997;40:124–9.

10. Saringer W, Nöbauer I, Reddy M, et al. Microsurgical anterior cervical foraminotomy (uncoforaminotomy) for unilateral radiculopathy: clinical results of a new technique. Acta Neurochir 2002;144:685–94.

Erratum

In Issue 42:3 of *Orthopedic Clinics*, the article entitled "Prognostic Factors and Outcome Measures in Perthes Disease" included a mislabeled figure. Figure 4 (page 306) is presented correctly below.

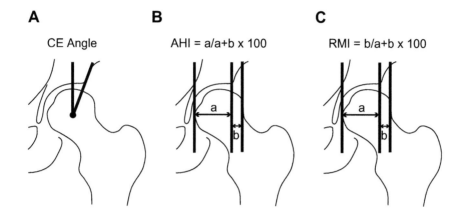

A CE Angle

B AHI = a/a+b x 100

C RMI = b/a+b x 100

DOI of original article: 10.1016/j.ocl.2011.03.004.

Orthop Clin N Am 43 (2012) 149
doi:10.1016/j.ocl.2011.10.003

Index

Note: Page numbers of article titles are in **boldface** type.

A

ACDF. *See* Anterior cervical diskectomy and fusion (ACDF)

Adjacent segment disease (ASD)
  after ACDF
    clinical evidence of, 54
    factors influencing, 55
  after cervical spinal fusion, **53–62**
    clinical evidence of, 54–56
    described, 53–54
    management of, **53–62**
      conservative options in, 57
      intraoperative preventive strategies in, 56–57
      preoperative prevention strategies in, 56
      principles of, 56–57
      surgical, 57–59
  after total disk replacement
    clinical evidence of, 55–56
  defined, 53
  revision cervical spine surgery for, 128

Anterior cervical diskectomy and fusion (ACDF)
  ASD after
    clinical evidence of, 54
    factors influencing, 55
  for complex CSM, 45
  incomplete
    revision cervical spine surgery for, 128–130
  vs. corpectomy
    for 2-level complex CSM, 44–45

Anterior cervical foraminotomy
  of cervical spine, 141–144

Arthritis
  rheumatoid
    C1-C2 posterior fixation in, 12

Arthroplasty
  disk
    revision cervical spine surgery for, 128–130

ASD. *See* Adjacent segment disease (ASD)

Atlantoaxial fusion
  esophageal and vertebral artery injuries during, 67–68

B

Bilateral foraminotomy
  of cervical spine
    approach and technique for, 139–141

C

C1-C2 posterior fixation, **11–18**
  anatomic considerations in, 11–12
  indications for, 12–13
  technique, 13–17
    C2 translaminar constructs in, 16–17
    dorsal writing in, 13
    polyaxial screw and rod fixation in, 14–16
    transarticular atlantoaxial arthrodesis in, 13–14

Carotid sheath
  anterior approach for complex CSM and, 43

Cerebrospinal fluid (CSF) leak
  surgical management of metastatic cervical spine tumors and, 82–84

Cervical spinal fusion
  ASD after, **53–62**. *See also* Adjacent segment disease (ASD), after cervical spinal fusion

Cervical spine
  degeneration in native and unfused
    clinical evidence of, 54–55

Cervical spine surgery
  complex
    esophageal and vertebral artery injuries during, **63–74**
      anterior surgery, 65–67
      atlantoaxial fusion, 67–68
      case example, 68–69
      subaxial posterior procedures, 67
  minimally invasive approaches, **137–147**
    anterior cervical foraminotomy, 141–144
    bilateral foraminotomy, 139–141
    case examples, 144–146
    contraindications to, 138
    described, 137–138
    indications for, 138
    lateral mass screw fixation, 139–141
    unilateral posterior foraminotomy, 138–139
  revision, **123–136**. *See also* Revision cervical spine surgery

Cervical spine trauma
  classification systems for
    SLIC, 90–92
    traditional, 89–90
  management of, **89–96**

Cervical spine tumors
  metastatic, **75–87**
    diagnosis of, 76–78

doi:10.1016/S0030-5898(11)00122-2
0030-5898/12/$ – see front matter © 2012 Elsevier Inc. All rights reserved